Fast Facts

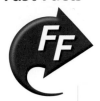

Fast Facts:

Parkinson's Disease

Second edition

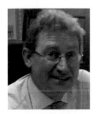

Christopher G Clough FRCP
Medical Director
King's College Hospital
London, UK

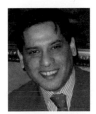

K Ray Chaudhuri MD FRCP DSc
Consultant Neurologist
National Parkinson Foundation Centre of Excellence
King's College Hospital and
University Hospital of Lewisham
London, UK

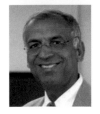

Kapil D Sethi MD FRCP
Professor of Neurology and
Director, Movement Disorders Program
Medical College of Georgia
Augusta, Georgia, USA

Collaborator: Sharon Muzerengi MBChB
Clinical Fellow in Neurology and Movement Disorders
University Hospital Lewisham, London

Declaration of Independence
This book is as balanced and as practical as we can make it.
Ideas for improvement are always welcome: feedback@fastfacts.com

HEALTH PRESS

Fast Facts: Parkinson's Disease
First published August 2003
Second edition April 2007

Health Press Limited, Elizabeth House, Queen Street, Abingdon,
Oxford OX14 3LN, UK
Tel: +44 (0)1235 523233
Fax: +44 (0)1235 523238

Book orders can be placed by telephone or via the website.
For regional distributors or to order via the website, please go to:
www.fastfacts.com
For telephone orders, please call +44 (0)1752 202301 (UK and Europe),
1 800 247 6553 (USA, toll free), +1 419 281 1802 (Americas) or
+61 (0)2 9351 6173 (Asia–Pacific).

Fast Facts is a trademark of Health Press Limited.

ISBN 978-1-905832-03-3

Clough CG (Christopher)
Fast Facts: Parkinson's Disease/
Christopher G Clough, K Ray Chaudhuri, Kapil D Sethi

Typesetting and page layout by Zed, Oxford, UK.
Printed by Fine Print (Services) Ltd, Oxford, UK.

Text printed with vegetable inks on fully biodegradable and
recyclable paper manufactured from sustainable forests.

444   001

Low emissions
during production

Low
chlorine

Sustainable
forests

Glossary

Apomorphine: drug that mimics dopamine, usually given by injection

Ballism: exaggerated involuntary movements leading to wild throwing gestures of the limbs (ballistic movements)

Bradykinesia (akinesia): slowness (absence) of movement

CAG expansion: trinucleotide repeat sequence of cytosine, adenosine and guanidine (there are over 35 CAG repeats in chromosome 4 in Huntington's disease)

Chorea: involuntary, fast bodily movements, usually affecting the distal limbs

Cogwheel rigidity: a rachet-like resistance or intermittent relaxation of tension under passive flexion, in the presence of tremor

COMT: catechol-O-methyl transferase; enzyme that metabolises levodopa and dopamine by 3-O-methylation

CT: computed tomography

DaTSCAN™: a diagnostic radiopharmaceutical, comprising radioiodine-labeled ioflupane (^{123}I) in an ethanolic solution, which is administered intravenously; the chemical binds with dopamine transporters in specific areas of the brain and shows up on single-photon emission tomography

Diphasic dyskinesia: abnormal movements that come on with the onset of levodopa response and recur as levodopa wears off

DLB: dementia with Lewy bodies; a progressive dementia, with hallucinations and fluctuating levels of attention

Doll's eye movement: the patient is asked to fixate straight ahead, and full eye movements are then demonstrated by moving the head (by flexion, extension and rotation)

Dopamine: neurotransmitter most depleted in Parkinson's disease

Dyskinesia: abnormal involuntary movements caused by drug treatment for Parkinson's disease

DZ: dizygotic; non-identical, from two fertilized eggs

Festination/festinating gait: characteristic gait of Parkinson's disease with small, hurrying steps, often accompanied by difficulty in gait initiation and sudden 'freezing' (stops and falls)

Fluorodopa: isotope-labeled neurotransmitter administered for positron emission tomography

GABA: γ-aminobutyric acid (4-aminobutanoic acid)

GDNF: glial-cell-line-derived neurotrophic factor

Lead-pipe rigidity: constant resistance to passive flexion, in the absence of tremor

Lewy bodies: intracytoplasmic neuronal inclusions found in the substantia nigra; pathological hallmark of Parkinson's disease

MPTP: 1-methyl-4-phenyl-1,2,3,6-tetrahydropyridine; by-product of pethidine synthesis produced illicitly and causing parkinsonism in drug addicts; now used to create animal models

MRI: magnetic resonance imaging; MRI of the skull characteristically shows no abnormality in Parkinson's disease

MSA: multiple-system atrophy; neuro-degenerative disorder characterized by symptoms causing slowness of movement, abnormal drop in blood pressure and bowel and bladder problems

MZ: monozygotic; identical, from one fertilized egg

Neuromelanin: pigment found within neurons

'On/off' syndrome: sudden fluctuation from an 'on' state (dyskinesia and reversal of parkinsonism) to an 'off' state (parkinsonism), secondary to levodopa treatment

Parkinsonism: the syndrome comprising rest-tremor, rigidity and bradykinesia

Parkinson's disease: the idiopathic variety of parkinsonism, usually responding to levodopa treatment and characterized pathologically by Lewy bodies

PDNS: Parkinson's disease nurse specialist

Peak-dose dyskinesia: abnormal movements that come on in the middle of levodopa response (usually related to the highest serum level of levodopa)

PET scan: brain image taken by positron emission tomography using radioactively labeled neurotransmitters or ligands

PSP: progressive supranuclear palsy; a rare neurodegenerative disorder that impairs movement and balance, with characteristic abnormalities of eye movements

RCT: randomized controlled trial

SALT: speech and language therapy

Serotonin (5-hydroxytryptamine, 5-HT): neurotransmitter important in maintaining equable mood

SPECT scan: single-photon emission computed tomography used for DaTSCAN™ analysis (a radiopharmaceutical used for the differential diagnosis of parkinsonian syndromes and essential tremor; *see* DaTSCAN™ above)

Sphincter electromyography: needle electrode test of the anal sphincter to detect loss of electrical activity in multiple-system atrophy

Stereotactic surgery: brain surgery performed through a small hole in the skull (burr or stereotaxy hole) using instruments attached to a stereotactic frame screwed to the skull

Striatum: basal ganglia nuclei comprising the caudate nucleus and putamen

Substantia nigra: black substance in the midbrain containing pigmented dopaminergic neurons

Thalamus: main sensorimotor nucleus, adjacent to the third ventricle

UPDRS: Unified Parkinson's Disease Rating Scale

Wilson's disease: early-onset dystonic condition caused by abnormal copper metabolism

Introduction

Parkinson's disease, first described by James Parkinson in 1817 (Figure 1), is one of the most important disabling illnesses of later life. It is estimated to affect 1% of 70-year-olds, but is also seen in younger people, with 10% of cases occurring before the age of 50.

The disease has become the pathfinder for other neurodegenerative disorders, since discovery of dopamine deficiency within the basal ganglia led to the development of the first effective treatment for a progressive neurodegenerative condition. Dopamine replacement therapy substantially reduces the symptoms of Parkinson's disease in most patients, improving their quality of life and initially appearing to decrease mortality.

Since the first edition of this book there have been many advances in the diagnosis and management of Parkinson's disease and in the care available for individuals with the condition. New genes have been described, and new methods to aid diagnosis such as transcranial ultrasound have been developed. Exciting developments in therapy, such as human fetal-cell transplantation or therapy with glial-cell-line-derived neurotrophic factor, now need thorough reassessment. Meanwhile, the therapeutic armamentarium continues to expand, with the licensing of rasagaline, rotigotine (the first transdermal-patch dopamine agonist) and intrajejunal infusion of levodopa to treat Parkinson's disease.

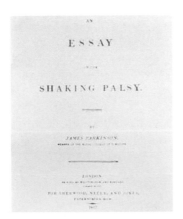

Figure 1 *An Essay on the Shaking Palsy* by James Parkinson (1817).

Guidelines highlighting the important role of multidisciplinary care have been published, while the focus of research has shifted from a bias towards motor symptoms to non-motor symptoms, with the publication of specific tools to assess and flag these important problems.

Although it is difficult to measure the specific economic cost of Parkinson's disease, studies suggest that the illness adversely affects the health-related quality of life of patients and imposes a significant economic burden on society comparable to that of other chronic conditions such as congestive heart failure, diabetes and stroke. Non-motor symptoms such as visual hallucinations, dementia and falls cause hospitalization and institutionalization, and have a major impact on the cost of the illness. Depression has been identified as one of the key symptoms of the illness. The annual direct cost of managing patients with Parkinson's disease at home is estimated at £4189; the cost rises to £19 338 for full-time institutionalization. Furthermore, the total direct cost of Parkinson's disease in patients in 'good health' is three times lower than for those in 'poor health'. These figures do not take into account hidden indirect costs such as loss of income from premature retirement, both for the patient and carer.

Given the burdens that Parkinson's disease can impose, we hope that this book will provide doctors, nurses and therapists with the latest information in order to improve as much as possible the lives of patients with Parkinson's disease and related disorders.

Key references

Findley L, Aujla M, Bain PG et al. Direct economic impact of Parkinson's disease: a research survey in the United Kingdom. *Mov Disord* 2003;18:1139–45.

Global Parkinson's Disease Survey Steering Committee. Factors impacting on quality of life in Parkinson's disease: results from an international survey. *Mov Disord* 2002;17:60–7.

Schrag A, Jahanshahi M, Quinn N. What contributes to quality of life in patients with Parkinson's disease? *J Neurol Neurosurg Psychiatry* 2000;69:308–12.

WHO. Parkinson's disease. In: *Neurological Disorders. Public Health Challenges.* World Health Organization, 2006:140–50. www.who.int/mental_health/neurology/ neurological_disorders_report_web.pdf

Epidemiology, pathophysiology and genetics

Epidemiology

Parkinson's disease is one of the most common neurodegenerative diseases, but estimating its incidence and prevalence is problematic, since there is no 'in-life' marker for idiopathic Parkinson's disease; the diagnosis can only be made with certainty if Lewy bodies (intracytoplasmic accumulations of protein in the brain) are found in the substantia nigra after death (see pages 12–13). Case ascertainment in community studies is difficult, and often other parkinsonian syndromes may be included.

Incidence and prevalence. Incidence is defined as the number of new cases in a specified time frame, and is not modified by factors affecting survival. Estimates of the annual incidence of Parkinson's disease are in the range of 4–20 per 100 000 individuals. The variability is accounted for by differences in the populations studied and by inclusion or exclusion of other clinical entities, such as essential tremor.

Prevalence is defined as the total number of cases in a given population at one time. A widely accepted figure for the prevalence of Parkinson's disease is approximately 200 per 100 000 population. In the USA, it is estimated that between 750 000 and 1.5 million people have the disease. In the UK, there are approximately 120 000–130 000 diagnosed cases, but there may be many more that remain undiagnosed.

Age, sex and ethnicity. Both the incidence and prevalence of Parkinson's disease increase with age, and the prevalence may be as high as 1 in 50 for patients over the age of 80 years. Men are 1.5 times more likely than women to develop the condition. Hospital-based studies have suggested that Parkinson's disease is less common in the black population.

Mortality. In 1967, Hoehn and Yahr published the first mortality study of Parkinson's disease in the pre-levodopa era. They found that up to 61% of patients were severely disabled or dead after 5–9 years of follow-up, which increased to more than 80% in those followed up for more than 10 years. Overall, mortality was three times that expected in the general population. In more than 20 reports on Parkinson's disease and mortality, two reported a rate of less than 1.5 compared with the general population: 11 reported mortality of 1.5–2, while the others reported rates greater than 2.

Several researchers have suggested that disability and mortality in Parkinson's disease show a sex difference, with significantly greater female mortality. However, there are other studies suggesting a poorer prognosis in men. Berger reported mortality of 3.1 for men and 1.8 for women, although these figures are much higher than the mortality reported in other studies. A recent study by Japanese investigators suggested a mean age of 71.9 years in men and 74.2 for women. In Japan, female patients appear to lose approximately 7 years of longevity compared with men once Parkinson's disease is diagnosed.

Although some would say that the life expectancy of patients with Parkinson's disease appears to have been prolonged, their lifespan is still probably less than that of the general population, as indicated in the Japanese study. The cause is complex. Improved survival is thought to be a result of the introduction of effective symptomatic therapy such as levodopa, while decreased or delayed mortality from comorbidity may partly account for the decreased mortality in younger people. Studies have suggested that relative survival for people with Parkinson's disease diagnosed before the age of 60 is similar to that for the general population, but for those who are older at diagnosis relative survival is less than expected .

The confusion regarding mortality in Parkinson's disease may be partly because the disease itself is not a primary or direct cause of death. In the USA, the average annual age-adjusted Parkinson's disease mortality between 1962 and 1984 was estimated as 2 deaths per 100 000 for white men and 1 death per 100 000 for non-white men, 1 death per 100 000 for white women and less than 1 death per 100 000 for non-white women. Mortality increased for persons aged 75 years and older, but declined for those younger than 70 years. Overall, published evidence suggests that mortality for Parkinson's disease increases in the older age groups but decreases for younger ages. The cause of death in Parkinson's disease is most commonly a secondary comorbid disorder. A Japanese study showed that the most common cause of death for all patients, regardless of age, was pneumonia.

Pathology

The main pathological feature of Parkinson's disease is the degeneration of neuromelanin-containing neurons in the pars compacta of the substantia nigra (Figure 1.1). Examination with the naked eye reveals pallor of this area, which is confirmed microscopically by a marked decrease in the number of neuromelanin-containing cells and the presence of Lewy bodies in the remaining nigral neurons.

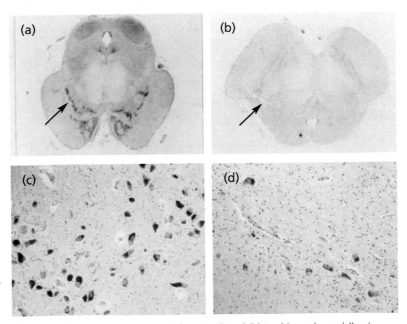

Figure 1.1 Sections through a (a) normal and (b) parkinsonian midbrain showing a characteristic loss of pigmentation in the substantia nigra (arrowed). Micrographs of the substantia nigra reveal (c) normal pigmented neurons in a normal brain and (d) the loss of pigmented neurons in a brain affected by Parkinson's disease.

Degeneration of pigmented neurons in the brainstem is not limited to the nigra but extends to the locus ceruleus and the dorsal motor nucleus of the vagus.

Lewy bodies are intracytoplasmic eosinophilic inclusions, which are typically found in the neurons of the substantia nigra (Figure 1.2). Neurites are tiny projections growing from the neurons, and Lewy bodies found within these projections are referred to as Lewy neurites. Lewy bodies are a pathological hallmark of idiopathic Parkinson's disease and are also found in other neurodegenerative diseases, such as dementia with Lewy bodies and Alzheimer's disease. Electron microscopy reveals that Lewy bodies are composed of filamentous material arranged in circular and linear profiles, sometimes radiating from an electron-dense core. Lewy bodies stain positively for ubiquitin and α-synuclein.

Lewy neurites are more widespread than well-delineated Lewy bodies. This has led to a re-examination of how Parkinson's disease pathology evolves. After examining a large number of brains, both clinically normal and with Parkinson's disease, Braak et al. suggested that the disease begins in the olfactory system and the dorsal vagal nucleus (stage 1), spreads to the nuclei of the caudal brainstem (the locus

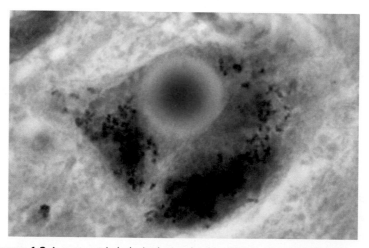

Figure 1.2 A concentric halo-inclusion body within a pigmented neuron. The presence of these Lewy bodies is characteristic of Parkinson's disease.

ceruleus and other nuclei; stage 2), then involves the substantia nigra in the middle stages of the disease (stage 3), and finally spreads to the cortex (stages 4 to 6). However, it must be emphasized that the Braak classification is based on Lewy-body formation and not on neuronal degeneration.

This and other clinical studies indicate that Parkinson's disease is a very complex disorder and that the motor manifestations required to make a diagnosis are just the tip of the iceberg.

Neuronal degeneration. The cause of neuronal degeneration in Parkinson's disease is unknown. The susceptible neurons are located in astroglial-poor regions such as the ventral tier. Glia may offer neuroprotection by providing neurotrophic factors that prevent cell death. Several hypotheses for neuronal degeneration have been proposed, including:
- oxidative stress, induced by dopamine metabolism or other factors
- defective mitochondrial energy metabolism
- excitotoxin- and xenobiotic-related cell death
- programmed cell death (apoptosis).

Oxidative stress. Free radicals, produced by dopamine metabolism, may result in the production of hydrogen peroxide and very reactive hydroxyl radicals. These can injure the phospholipid layer of the cell membrane and induce apoptosis, and can also damage other molecules, such as DNA and proteins. Free radicals are scavenged by enzyme systems, including glutathione and superoxide dismutase.

Pathological studies have shown reduced glutathione levels in patients who died from Parkinson's disease, suggesting excessive utilization of glutathione by free radicals. Although there is some evidence that cell injury related to free radicals is implicated in Parkinson's disease, this is not certain. A free-radical scavenger, such as selegiline, has no definite effect on disease progression.

The substantia nigra contains high levels of iron. Free iron can induce decomposition of lipid and peroxide and formation of hydroxyl radicals. Iron levels are increased in brains affected by Parkinson's disease, as well as in other neurodegenerative disorders. This may, however, be secondary to neurodegeneration.

Defective mitochondrial energy metabolism. The study of the toxin 1-methyl-4-phenyl-1,2,3,6-tetrahydropyridine (MPTP) has afforded an insight into defects in mitochondrial energy metabolism in Parkinson's disease (Figure 1.3). Originally, MPP^+ (the active by-product of MPTP) was thought to damage dopaminergic neurons by production of free radicals, but subsequently it has been found that MPP^+ inhibits complex 1 (reduced nicotinamide adenine dinucleotide [NADH], coenzyme Q 1 reductase) in the mitochondrial energy cycle. The resulting paralysis of energy production may account for the degeneration of dopaminergic neurons in MPTP primate models as well as in humans developing symptoms resembling those of Parkinson's disease with MPTP. Many studies have found complex 1 defects in patients with Parkinson's disease.

Excitotoxin/xenobiotic metabolism. Defects in the enzymes that break down endogenous and exogenous chemicals (such as excitotoxins and xenobiotics, respectively) are seen in patients with Parkinson's disease. Several environmental toxins, including organochloropesticides, may be toxic to mitochondria. It is possible that these chemicals are not

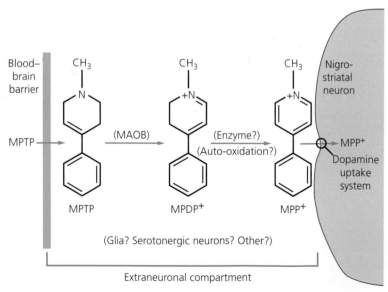

Figure 1.3 The metabolic fate of 1-methyl-4-phenyl-1,2,3,6-tetrahydro-pyridine (MPTP). MAOB, monoamine oxidase B.

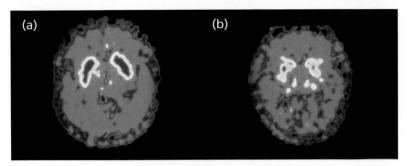

Figure 1.4 Positron emission tomography scans showing uptake of radio-labeled flurodopa by the basal ganglia in (a) a normal brain and (b) the brain of a patient with Parkinson's disease, in which the uptake is reduced.

metabolized effectively in such patients, which may account for susceptibility to the condition.

Nigral cell loss. There is gradual loss of pigmented neurons in the substantia nigra with age. It is estimated that approximately 70–80% of nigral neurons are lost before clinical symptoms of Parkinson's disease become apparent. However, on 6-fluorodopa positron emission tomography (PET) scans, the threshold appears to occur when approximately 50% of fluorodopa uptake is lost. This difference may reflect overactivity of the remaining nigral neurons in an effort to maintain nigrostriatal dopamine transmission (Figure 1.4).

Presymptomatic duration. There are several hypotheses concerning the length of the presymptomatic phase of Parkinson's disease.

- There may be a very long presymptomatic period, spanning 2 or 3 decades; it is even possible that a static insult at some point in a person's life may predispose them to develop Parkinson's disease because of the attrition of dopamine-bearing neurons with age.
- Microglial proliferation, found postmortem in people with Parkinson's disease, suggests ongoing neuronal death. This may mean the presymptomatic period is short.
- Longitudinal fluorodopa-uptake measurements demonstrate a short presymptomatic period. Fluorodopa uptake declines at a rate of about 10% per year in Parkinson's disease; the decline is most rapid in the early stages of the disease. The change is also more rapid in

akinetic-rigid patients than in those with tremor-dominant disease, and in patients with young-onset as opposed to old-age-onset Parkinson's disease. Accordingly, it is possible that the presymptomatic period is as short as 5–6 years.

Presymptomatic detection. Individuals with a family history of Parkinson's disease, and those with rapid eye movement (REM) behavior disorder and impaired olfaction, may have a higher risk of developing the disease. In the future, it may be possible to recognize individuals who are at risk and to initiate neuropreventative therapy. In a 2-year study, 10% of these high-risk individuals showed deterioration in dopaminergic markers, and some developed clinical disease.

Pathophysiology

Nigral degeneration results in loss of dopamine in the nigrostriatal tract. Nigrostriatal dopaminergic transmission influences motor function through a complex route involving parallel circuits, some of which are inhibitory while others are facilitatory (Figure 1.5). The final common pathway of movement is the motor unit that is influenced through many cortical, reticulospinal and corticospinal tracts. The striatum influences the supplementary motor area through its connections with the ventrolateral nucleus of the thalamus.

The striatal output uses γ-aminobutyric acid (GABA) and is entirely inhibitory. The striatum projects to the medial globus pallidus via two pathways, one indirect and the other direct. Dopamine is inhibitory to the indirect striatopallidal pathway, which first projects to the lateral globus pallidus. The lateral globus pallidus in turn sends another inhibitory projection to the subthalamic nucleus, using GABA as a neurotransmitter. The subthalamic nucleus sends an excitatory glutamatergic output to the medial globus pallidus. Dopamine is excitatory via the D_1 receptors to the direct striatopallidal pathway.

In Parkinson's disease there is a relative lack of dopamine, which leads to defective excitation of the direct circuit and, therefore, decreased GABA-mediated inhibition. This results in overactivity of the neurons of the medial globus pallidus. Also, because of the lack of dopamine there is defective D_2-mediated striatal inhibition (indirect pathway), accentuated striatal inhibition of the lateral pallidus and

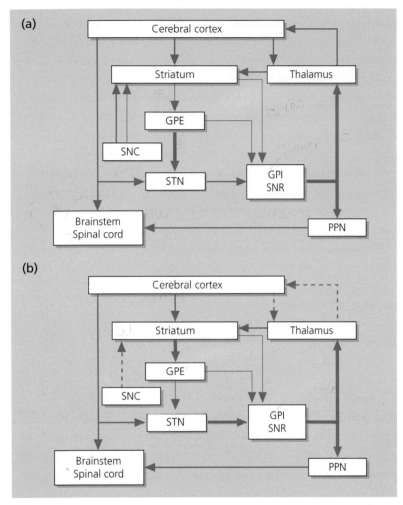

Figure 1.5 (a) The normal circuitry involved in the control of movement, in which the direct pathway (via the globus pallidus interna [(GPI]) and the indirect pathway (via the globus pallidus externa [GPE] and subthalamic nucleus [STN]) are in balance, producing optimal excitation of the thalamus and, thereafter, the cerebral cortex. (b) In Parkinson's disease, there is progressive loss of dopaminergic input from the substantia nigra (SNC) to the striatum, resulting in an imbalance between the direct and indirect pathways, with overactivity of the indirect pathway; overinhibition of the thalamus results in slow and reduced movement. PPN, pedunculopontine nucleus; SNR, substantia nigra reticulata.

17

disinhibition of the subthalamic nucleus because of the underactivity of GABAergic lateral-globus-pallidus outflow. The overactivity of the subthalamic nucleus then overexcites the medial globus pallidus.

The net result of both the direct and the indirect pathways in the absence of dopamine is overexcitation of the medial globus pallidus, leading to excessive inhibition of the thalamus. If the thalamus cannot excite the cerebral cortex, this leads to akinesia (absence of body movements) and other symptoms of Parkinson's disease.

While this model explains many of the signs and symptoms of Parkinson's disease, there are several inconsistencies. Pallidotomy ameliorates not only bradykinesia but also levodopa-induced dyskinesias; this is very hard to reconcile with the circuitry discussed here.

Also, in animal models of hemiballism (vigorous, involuntary movements on one side of the body), a lesion of the subthalamic nucleus results in contralateral hemiballism/hemichorea, which in turn can be abolished by a lesion of the medial globus pallidus.

Risk factors

Although Parkinson's disease was first described nearly 200 years ago, it is still impossible to define exactly which individuals are at risk. The aging process is intricately related to the development of Parkinson's disease but is not solely responsible, as some patients develop the disease early in life. Furthermore, the type of dopamine-cell loss in normal aging differs from that in Parkinson's disease. Certain personality traits and environmental factors may increase the risk of Parkinson's disease developing. People with a family history of Parkinson's disease are also at higher risk of developing the disease (see Genetics, pages 19–23).

Personality traits. Patients with certain personality traits, in particular those who are very disciplined and have a tendency to be shy and occasionally depressive, may have a higher risk of developing Parkinson's disease. Such patients usually do not abuse alcohol or cigarettes; it is possible that the apparent protective effects of smoking may be due to nicotine or other tobacco compounds. It is not clear whether these behavioral traits are a genuine risk factor or merely an early indication of dopamine deficiency.

Environmental factors implicated in the genesis of Parkinson's disease include toxins such as herbicides and pesticides (e.g. rotenone). A few studies have found consumption of well-water to be a risk factor, and Parkinson's disease seems to be more common in farming communities. Heavy metals, including manganese, have also been implicated; for example, exposure to the manganese found in welding fumes has been suggested as a risk factor (see below).

A theory for environmental causation was boosted when the use of an illicit drug, MPTP, a by-product of pethidine synthesis, resulted in a mini-epidemic of an illness similar to Parkinson's disease in young people who were abusing the drug intravenously. MPTP destroyed dopamine neurons in the substantia nigra of those affected. The condition responded to dopa drugs in the same way as Parkinson's disease, but Lewy-body inclusions were not detected postmortem.

Welding-related parkinsonism. Rare cases of parkinsonism have been linked with exposure to welding fumes, but there is no conclusive evidence that welding either causes parkinsonism or accelerates the onset of Parkinson's disease. Although a community study found higher rates of parkinsonism among welders, this and other such trials have had methodological flaws and the findings have not been replicated. Scandinavian and Korean studies among welders have not shown any relation between welding and Parkinson's disease.

Genetics

Genetic investigation of Parkinson's disease is complicated by the same factors that influence the study of its epidemiology. Up to 25% of cases diagnosed as idiopathic Parkinson's disease may actually be some other form of atypical parkinsonism. The familial patterns of Parkinson's disease can be masked if affected family members die before clinical signs become apparent. As Parkinson's disease usually manifests late in life, there are very few affected families with living members from more than two generations. Despite these limitations, significant progress has been made in our understanding of the genetics of the disease from familial aggregation studies, examination of large kindreds and studies in twins.

Familial risk. Individuals with a positive family history have twice the risk of developing Parkinson's disease symptoms. The risk for siblings is increased significantly if there is an affected sibling with young-onset Parkinson's disease. The risk increases further to 12–24% if both a sibling and a parent are affected.

Large kindred studies. Several families with Parkinson's disease or atypical parkinsonism have been described. A landmark study, initially reported by Golbe et al., of a family who had migrated to New Jersey, USA, from Contursi, Italy, suggested an autosomal-dominant inheritance pattern with high penetrance (i.e. a high frequency of Parkinson's disease among family members with the same genotype). There has been pathological confirmation of Lewy bodies in some family members. Genetic linkage studies showed that the abnormal gene *PARK1* is located on chromosome 4q21–23 (Table 1.1) and encodes the protein α-synuclein. Subsequently, the mutation was found to be a substitution of threonine for alanine. How the mutation leads to nigral degeneration and Lewy-body formation is unclear. Lewy bodies stain positively for α-synuclein, and α-synuclein aggregation leads to fibril formation. Wszolek et al. identified another large family with 18 affected members within four generations. The gene for this kindred, *PARK3*, has been mapped to chromosome 2p13.

However, the *PARK1* and *PARK3* mutations have not been found in many families with autosomal-dominant Parkinson's disease or sporadic Parkinson's disease. Other mutations are being discovered elsewhere (Table 1.1); mutation of the *DJ1* gene linked to autosomal-recessive early-onset Parkinson's disease, known as *PARK7*, was identified in a Dutch and an Italian family, while *PARK8*, with a locus on chromosome 12, was identified in a Japanese family.

Autosomal-recessive juvenile parkinsonism has been studied mainly in Japan. The gene locus for juvenile parkinsonism has been mapped to chromosome 6q and named *Parkin*. The same mutation has been found in European families in individuals with juvenile or young-onset Parkinson's disease. This gene has a 30% homology with the gene that encodes ubiquitin, and is expressed in various regions of the brain (including the substantia nigra) and in liver, heart,

TABLE 1.1

Some genes implicated in inherited parkinsonism

Symbol	Inheritance	Product	Location	Gene
PARK1	AD	α-synuclein*	4q21.3–q23	SNCA
PARK2	AR, juvenile onset	Parkin	6q25.2–q27	Parkin
PARK3	AD, Lewy body	Unknown	2p13	–
PARK4	AD, Lewy body	Unknown	4p15	–
PARK5	AD	UCHL1	4p14	UCHL1
PARK6	AR, early onset	PINK	1p35–p36	PINK1
PARK7	AR, early onset	DJ1 protein	1p36	DJ1
PARK8	AD	Dardarin†	12p11.2–q13.1	LRRK2
PARK9	AR	Unknown	1p36	–
PARK10		Unknown	unspecified	–
PARK11		Unknown	2q36	–

*Non-A4 component of amyloid precursor.
†Derived from the Basque word *dardar*, meaning 'tremor'.
AD, autosomal-dominant; AR, autosomal-recessive; LRRK, leucine-rich repeat kinase; PINK, phosphatase and tensin homolog (PTEN)-induced putative kinase; SNCA, α-synuclein; UCHL1, ubiquitin carboxy-terminal hydrolase L1; –, gene yet to be cloned.

testis and skeletal muscle. Parkin protein is a ubiquitin ligase involved in protein degradation. The *Parkin* mutation appears to lead to defective protein ubiquination, leading to protein aggregation and cell death.

Recent findings in the genetics of Parkinson's disease include the identification of the leucine-rich repeat kinase 2 (*LRRK2*) gene mutation. LRRK2 is part of the family of *Roco* genes, and it encodes for the protein dardarin. *LRRK2* has been associated with familial late-onset Parkinson's disease and a few cases of sporadic late-onset Parkinson's disease. The phenotype appears to be identical to sporadic

21

Parkinson's disease, but is associated with behavioral disorders, leg tremor and little cognitive decline. Recently, one case of the *LRRK2* mutation (Ile1371Val substitution) was reported, with the typical Lewy-body pathology, staining positive for ubiquitin and α-synuclein, identical to idiopathic sporadic Parkinson's disease.

Previously identified genes have been pivotal to understanding the process of neurodegeneration. However, the clinical impact of these genes has been limited because they are usually identified in patients with early-onset Parkinson's disease (e.g with the *Parkin* and *PINK1* [phosphatase and tensin homolog (PTEN)-induced putative kinase 1] genes) or with atypical parkinsonism (as with the *MAPT* [microtubule-associated protein Tau] gene).

Gly2019Ser is the most common *LRRK2* substitution, accounting for 0.5–2% of apparently 'sporadic' cases and about 5% of familial cases. This substitution is identified more frequently in North African Arabs and Ashkenazi Jews.

In the recent genome-wide scan for Parkinson's disease (GenePD) study, which investigated the effect of heterozygous *Parkin* mutations on age of onset in patients with familial Parkinson's disease, one member from each of 183 families was screened for *PARK2* mutations: 12.6% of the families were positive. Of these, 43% were compound heterozygotes, 13% were homozygotes and 10% were heterozygotes. The age of onset of Parkinson's disease was significantly lower in those with one *Parkin* mutation than in those with none (11.7 years earlier), and also significantly lower in those with two mutations than in those with one (13.2 years earlier). The study showed that the *Parkin* mutation is not rare, and that heterozygosity significantly lowers the age of onset of Parkinson's disease.

Studies in twins have been performed since 1967. Ward et al. studied 43 monozygotic (MZ) and 19 dizygotic (DZ) pairs of twins, and found that the concordance rate for parkinsonism was no more frequent in twins than expected, given the general rate of disease. They concluded that the main causative factors are probably not genetic. However, Parkinson's disease may be asymptomatic in the unaffected twin. Burn et al. studied 18-fluorodopa PET scans in sets of twins in which one of each pair had clinical Parkinson's disease. The clinically unaffected twin frequently had abnormally low 18-fluorodopa uptake. Follow-up of some of the twins revealed worsening of this abnormality, suggesting progressive deterioration of nigrostriatal function. The PET findings suggested concordance rates of 45% for MZ and 29% for DZ twins. Therefore, it seems that a substantial genetic contribution to Parkinson's disease is likely.

Key points – epidemiology, pathophysiology and genetics

- Parkinson's disease is one of the most common neuro-degenerative diseases, with a prevalence of approximately 200 per 100 000 population.
- The incidence and prevalence of Parkinson's disease increases sharply with age.
- Men are 1.5 times more likely than women to develop the disease.
- Pathologically, Parkinson's disease is characterized by degeneration of neuromelanin-containing neurons, presenting as pallor of the substantia nigra; Lewy bodies in the remaining nigral neurons are a pathological hallmark of the disease after death.
- The cause of neuronal degeneration is uncertain.
- Braak has suggested that the condition may begin in the olfactory bundle and lower brainstem, and studies are under way to detect Parkinson's disease at a premotor phase.
- A shy or depressive personality, exposure to environmental toxins or heavy metals and a positive family history of the condition are all risk factors for Parkinson's disease.

Key references

Berger K, Breteler MM, Helmer C et al. Prognosis with Parkinson's disease in Europe: a collaborative study of population-based cohorts. Neurologic Diseases in the Elderly Research Group. *Neurology* 2000;54(suppl 5):S24–7.

Braak H, Ghebremedhin E, Rub U et al. Stages in the development of Parkinson's disease-related pathology. *Cell Tissue Res* 2004;318:121–34.

Burn DJ, Mark MH, Playford ED et al. Parkinson's disease in twins studied with 18F-dopa and positron emission tomography. *Neurology* 1992;42:1894–900.

Diamond SG, Markham CH, Hoehn MM et al. Effect of age at onset on progression and mortality in Parkinson's disease. *Neurology* 1989;39:1187–90.

Foltynie T, Sawcer S, Brayne C, Barker RA. The genetic basis of Parkinson's disease. *J Neurol Neurosurg Psychiatry* 2002;73: 363–70.

Giordana MT, D'Agostino C, Albani G et al. Neuropathology of Parkinson's disease associated with the *LRRK2* Ile1371Val mutation. *Mov Disord* 2007;22:275–8.

Golbe LI, Di Iorio G, Sanges G et al. Clinical genetic analysis of Parkinson's disease in the Contursi kindred. *Ann Neurol* 1996;40: 767–75.

Hely MA, Morris JG, Reid WG et al. Age at onset: the major determinant of outcome in Parkinson's disease. *Acta Neurol Scand* 1995;92:455–63.

Hoehn MM, Yahr MD. Parkinsonism: onset, progression, and mortality. *Neurology* 1998;50:318 (reprinted from *Neurology* 1967;17:427–42).

Khan NL, Jain S, Lynch JM et al. Mutations in the gene *LRRK2* encoding dardarin (*PARK8*) cause familial Parkinson's disease: clinical, pathological, olfactory and functional imaging and genetic data. *Brain* 2005;128:2786–96.

Mata IF, Ross OA, Kachergus J et al. *LRRK2* mutations are a common cause of Parkinson's disease in Spain. *Eur J Neurol* 2006;13:391–4.

Ponsen MM, Stoffers D, Booij J et al. Idiopathic hyposmia as a preclinical sign of Parkinson's disease. *Ann Neurol* 2004;56:173–81.

Sun M, Latourelle JC, Wooten GF et al. Influence of heterozygosity for *Parkin* mutation on onset age in familial Parkinson disease: the GenePD study. *Arch Neurol* 2006; 63:826–32.

Ward CD, Duvoisin RC, Ince SE et al. Parkinson's disease in 65 pairs of twins and in a set of quadruplets. *Neurology* 1983;33:815–24.

Wszolek ZK, Pfeiffer B, Fulgham JR et al. Western Nebraska family (family D) with autosomal dominant parkinsonism. *Neurology* 1995;45: 502–5.

When, in 1817, James Parkinson first described the features of paralysis agitans in six patients, he did not refer to the typical cogwheel rigidity, and mistook bradykinesia for paralysis. Nevertheless, his description of the tremor, posture (Figure 2.1) and clinical course of the disease has hardly been improved. Most cases of Parkinson's disease are easily recognizable at an early stage, but many are missed if tremor is absent; gradual slowing in performance may be instead attributed to aging or aches and pains, and loss of function may be ascribed to other causes.

Parkinsonism is a clinical syndrome (Table 2.1) and may have a number of causes. When the condition appears to be idiopathic, and, in particular, responds to levodopa therapy, it is referred to as Parkinson's disease.

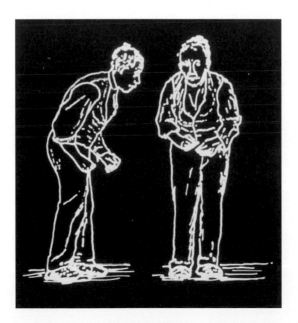

Figure 2.1 *Paralysis agitans,* as first depicted by James Parkinson. The characteristic fixed posture is shown.

TABLE 2.1

Diagnosis of parkinsonism

Essential features
- Bradykinesia and
  - tremor (resting) and/or
  - rigidity (cogwheel or lead-pipe; see page 29)

Additional features
- Postural imbalance
- Fixed, stooped posture
- Dystonic postures, e.g. striatal hand
- Hypomimia ('masked' face)
- Shuffling, short-step gait (with or without festination)
- Freezing episodes (sometimes known as paradoxical akinesia)
- Seborrhea of the scalp
- Constipation
- Bladder symptoms (sometimes known as pseudoprostatism)
- Bulbar symptoms
  - dysarthria
  - dysphagia
- Pain
- Mental and cognitive disturbance

Early indicators

Signs may be subtle in the early stages of the disease. In suspected cases it is often helpful to ask patients what tasks they find difficult.
- Dressing may become awkward and take longer than usual.
- Eating and swallowing may slow down (with others assuming that the affected person has a poor appetite and not allowing enough time for meals).
- Walking in crowds may be difficult, because the person cannot make the rapid adjustments necessary to avoid bumping into other people.

- Getting out of a low chair can be problematic (although the patient may have noticed this, they may be unable to explain why it is difficult).
- Handwriting often deteriorates, with the writing typically becoming smaller; if the patient is asked to draw a spiral this will be smaller than that drawn by the doctor or nurse in the clinic (Figure 2.2). Comparison of the patient's writing from the past with that drawn in the clinic may be useful.
- Facial expression becomes impassive and the patient may blink infrequently; this mask-like expression can conceal the patient's normal thoughts and emotions.
- Speech may be soft and low in volume, with frequent pauses. Patients may have difficulty enunciating syllables and words separately, so the sounds become merged and speech may be difficult to understand.

Symptoms and signs

Tremor is rhythmic shaking and involuntary movement of part(s) of the body as a result of repetitive muscle contractions. The presence of an obvious tremor often leads both patients and their carers to suspect Parkinson's disease. Parkinsonian tremor is worse at rest (4–7 Hz) and is often unilateral. It affects 70% of patients with Parkinson's disease and is the presenting feature in most cases. However, those presenting with akinetic-rigid parkinsonism may never have tremor.

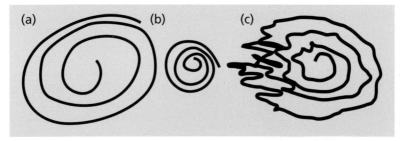

Figure 2.2 Spiral drawings may help to differentiate between parkinsonian and essential tremor. When asked to replicate a spiral (a) drawn by the doctor or nurse, a patient with (b) parkinsonian tremor is likely to produce a much smaller version, whereas a patient with (c) essential tremor will produce a shakier but similar-sized version of the original.

Tremor often has a rotary component that is almost always indicative of Parkinson's disease; for example, patients may be seen 'pill rolling', the action of rolling a small sphere between thumb and index finger.

Parkinsonian vs essential tremor. Parkinsonian tremor does not interfere with activity, whereas essential tremor is postural and affects function, such as carrying a cup of tea.

It is important to differentiate essential tremor from parkinsonian tremor (see Figure 2.2), as the former carries a more benign prognosis and is twice as common, with a prevalence of at least 400 per 100 000 (Table 2.2). Parkinsonian tremor, while worrying and

TABLE 2.2

Comparison of parkinsonian tremor and essential tremor

Feature	Parkinsonian tremor	Essential tremor
Age at onset	Usually > 50 years	> 10 years
Occurrence	Incidence increases with each decade of age	Incidence remains the same with each decade of age
Family history	Rare	Common
Site	Usually hands, also legs and jaw; head uncommon	Hands, head (a no–no or yes–yes motion), vocal
Characteristics	At rest; reduced by supination/pronation action; increased by mental concentration	Postural; increased by flexion/extension action; diminished by mental concentration
Frequency (Hz)	4–7	8–12
Lead-pipe rigidity*	Yes	No
Cogwheel rigidity*	Yes	Rare
Alcohol	No effect	Often improves
Treatment	Dopaminergics, anticholinergics	β-blockers, primidone

*See definitions, page 29.

embarrassing for the patient, is generally a good sign in Parkinson's disease, although it will only partially respond to dopaminergic therapy.

Bradykinesia/akinesia is difficulty in initiating, and slowness in executing, movement. It is the most disabling motor sign of Parkinson's disease. It first affects fine movements such as fastening buttons, and handwriting that starts normal sized, becomes smaller and more cramped, and may progressively tail off (micrographia). One or both arms may stop swinging when walking.

Later, gait is affected, with difficulty starting off walking, small steps and shuffling. 'Festination' describes the typical hurrying gait, which may be interrupted by sudden stops as if the patient is nailed to the floor. Carers may nudge patients to start them moving again. These freezing episodes (paroxysmal akinesia) are often provoked by visual stimuli, such as an open doorway, or by anxiety. Many patients develop tricks to overcome the symptom, such as stepping over an inverted walking stick or marching to a rhythm. Eventually, patients may need a wheelchair; however, if one is necessary in the early stages of disease, the diagnosis should be reappraised.

Other signs of bradykinesia include characteristic facial impassivity (hypomimia), which, if unilateral, may be misinterpreted as facial paralysis. Bradykinetic laryngeal movement leads to quiet, monotonous speech that may tail off in volume.

Rigidity is often detected by physicians. Patients complain of muscular stiffness and pain, which may be diffuse or localized to one limb or the trunk. Parkinsonian rigidity is detected by moving the body part slowly and gently (in contrast to the quick movement needed to elicit clasp-knife rigidity of pyramidal origin).

Parkinsonian rigidity, which can be activated by performing mirror movements in the opposite limb, presents as one of two types:
- 'lead-pipe' rigidity – a constant resistance to passive movement, in the absence of tremor.
- 'cogwheel' rigidity – a superimposed clicking resistance like a ratchet, in the presence of tremor.

Postural problems. The bent posture of Parkinson's disease is probably due to rigidity and muscle spasm, although other factors may contribute.

Flexion is encountered particularly in the neck and trunk, and also when the arms are brought forward in front of the body. Additional flexion at the hips and knees may lead to walking on tiptoe (simian gait) in fully developed disease.

Postural imbalance can be detected by the 'pull' test. The doctor stands behind the patient and applies a quick pull backwards to the front of the shoulders. Parkinsonian patients typically fall backwards or totter without corrective action, leading to a fall 'en bloc' (in one piece).

Falls are common in late Parkinson's disease and are a major cause of morbidity. They may be due to postural imbalance, a displaced centre of gravity and/or failure to detect displacement and take corrective action.

Non-motor symptom complex. A wide range of non-motor symptoms (NMS) have been described in Parkinson's disease, all of which are likely to have a major effect on the health-related quality of life of patients. These symptoms include depression, dementia, sleep disorders, bowel and bladder problems, fatigue, apathy, pain and autonomic dysfunction (Table 2.3). NMS are common and can occur at all stages of the disease, even before the diagnosis (premotor phase).

Non-motor symptom complex has been poorly recognized by healthcare professionals, as there is a tendency to concentrate on motor symptoms. However the recent development and validation of instruments such as the NMS questionnaire (NMSQuest; Table 2.4), scale (NMSS) and the revised Unified Parkinson's Disease Rating Scale (MDS-UPDRS, in development) is likely to make comprehensive evaluation of NMS in patients with Parkinson's disease possible.

Confirmation of diagnosis

There are as yet no specific tests for the diagnosis of Parkinson's disease. Challenge tests, as discussed on pages 33–4, are not routinely recommended for diagnostic purposes in the recently published guidelines by the UK's National Institute for Health and Clinical Excellence, but guidelines vary worldwide.

TABLE 2.3

The non-motor symptom complex

Neuropsychiatric symptoms
- Depression, apathy, anxiety
- Anhedonia
- Attention deficit
- Hallucinations, illusion, delusions
- Dementia
- Obsessional behavior (usually drug induced), repetitive behavior
- Confusion
- Delirium (could be drug induced)
- Panic attacks

Sleep disorders
- Restless legs and periodic limb movements
- REM behavior disorder and REM loss of atonia
- Non-REM sleep-related movement disorders
- Excessive daytime somnolence
- Vivid dreaming
- Insomnia
- Sleep-disordered breathing

Sensory symptoms
- Pain
- Paresthesia
- Olfactory disturbance

Autonomic symptoms
- Bladder disturbances
  - Urgency
  - Nocturia
  - Frequency
- Sweating
- Orthostatic hypotension (OH)
  - Falls related to OH
  - Coat-hanger pain*
- Sexual dysfunction
    Hypersexuality (likely to be drug induced)
  - Erectile dysfunction
- Dry eyes (xerostomia)

Gastrointestinal symptoms†
- Dribbling of saliva
- Ageusia (loss of taste)
- Dysphagia/choking
- Reflux, vomiting
- Nausea
- Constipation
- Unsatisfactory voiding of bowel
- Fecal incontinence

Other symptoms
- Fatigue
- Diplopia
- Blurred vision
- Seborrhea
- Weight loss
- Weight gain (possibly drug induced)

*A rare type of pain that occurs at the back of the head and neck and across the shoulder muscles.
†Overlap with autonomic symptoms.
REM, rapid eye movement.

TABLE 2.4

Questions to ask in the assessment of non-motor symptoms

Have you experienced any of the following during the past month?*

	Yes	No
• Dribbling of saliva during the daytime	☐	☐
• Loss, or change in, your ability to taste or smell	☐	☐
• Difficulty swallowing food or drink, or problems with choking	☐	☐
• Vomiting or feelings of sickness	☐	☐
• Constipation (less than three bowel movements per week), or having to strain to pass a stool	☐	☐
• Fecal incontinence	☐	☐
• Feeling that your bowel emptying is incomplete	☐	☐
• A sense of urgency to pass urine	☐	☐
• Getting up regularly at night to pass urine	☐	☐
• Unexplained pains (not due to known conditions, e.g. arthritis)	☐	☐
• Unexplained change in weight (not due to a change in diet)	☐	☐
• Problems remembering things that have happened recently, or forgetting to do things	☐	☐
• Loss of interest in what is happening around you, or in doing things	☐	☐
• Seeing/hearing things that you know, or are told, are not there	☐	☐
• Difficulty concentrating or staying focused	☐	☐
• Feeling sad, 'low' or 'blue'	☐	☐
• Feeling anxious, frightened or panicky	☐	☐
• Feeling less, or more, interested in sex	☐	☐
• Finding it difficult to have sex (when you try)	☐	☐
• Feeling light-headed, dizzy or weak when standing up from sitting or lying	☐	☐
• Falling	☐	☐
• Finding it difficult to stay awake during activities (e.g working, driving or eating)	☐	☐

CONTINUED

TABLE 2.4 (CONTINUED)

	Yes	No
• Finding it difficult to get to sleep, or to stay asleep, at night	☐	☐
• Intense, vivid dreams or frightening dreams	☐	☐
• Talking or moving about during your sleep as if you are 'acting' out a dream	☐	☐
• Unpleasant sensations in your legs at night or while resting, and a feeling that you need to move	☐	☐
• Swelling of your legs	☐	☐
• Excessive sweating	☐	☐
• Double vision	☐	☐
• Believing things are happening to you that other people say are not true	☐	☐

*Patients should be asked to answer 'yes' if they have experienced the symptom during the past month, but to answer 'no' if they have experienced the problem but not in the past month.

Adapted from the Parkinson's Disease (PD) Non-Motor Symptoms Questionnaire (NMSQuest), developed and validated by the International PD Non-Motor Group. (Available online at http://tinyurl.com/286.xfp). © Parkinson's Disease Society 2006.

Dopaminergic challenge. The response to levodopa, or to dopaminergic agents such as apomorphine, can be used to assess accuracy of diagnosis, management and prognosis of the parkinsonian patient. Diagnostic issues can be assessed either after a single challenge or following conventional dopa treatment monitored over several weeks (Table 2.5). However, there is some concern about the use of levodopa in untreated, levodopa-naïve patients, since a possible priming action of levodopa for the development of future dyskinesias has been demonstrated in animal models.

Patients with idiopathic Parkinson's disease will show a significant response to dopaminergic agents; indeed, about 50% of patients will go on to develop dyskinesia after 5 years of standard therapy with levodopa (at doses exceeding 600 mg/day), although this proportion is lower when smaller doses of levodopa (150–300 mg/day) are given.

TABLE 2.5

Dopaminergic challenge*

An improvement of ≥ 20% in the Parkinson's disease score[†] after one of the following challenges strongly suggests Parkinson's disease

Either

- Give three doses of domperidone,[‡] 20 mg orally, in 24 hours
- Measure Parkinson's disease score
- Give one dose of levodopa, 250 mg orally
- Measure Parkinson's disease score again 2 hours later

Or

- Give three doses of domperidone,[‡] 20 mg orally, in 24 hours
- Measure Parkinson's disease score
- Give apomorphine, 3 mg subcutaneously
- Measure Parkinson's disease score again 20 minutes later

*Not routinely recommended by the UK's National Institute for Health and Clinical Excellence for differentiating between parkinsonian syndromes. This, however, is not the advice in all countries; national guidelines should be consulted. Guidelines issued by the American Academy of Neurology do recommend challenge tests as good 'level B' evidence for confirmation of diagnosis.

[†]Disease scores should be measured using the Unified Parkinson's Disease Rating Scale (UPDRS) or the SCale for Outcomes in PArkinson's disease (SCOPA)-Motor scale. The UPDRS is being revised; a new version endorsed by the Movement Disorder Society (MDS-UPDRS), incorporating a non-motor section, will be available after validation (see www.mdvu.org/pdf/updrs.pdf).

[‡]Domperidone is not routinely available in the USA, and use of vestibular sedatives or metoclopramide may be hazardous because of central dopamine blocking and other extrapyramidal side effects. Antiemetics such as nabilone or ondansetron (although expensive) may be used instead.

Approximately 20% of patients with parkinsonian symptoms exhibit little response to dopaminergic treatment. Many of these have a different underlying disease, such as multiple-system atrophy (MSA), progressive supranuclear palsy (PSP), corticobasal degeneration or primary striatonigral degeneration (Table 2.6). Patients who do not respond to levodopa therapy have a worse prognosis, probably with a progressive course and reduced life expectancy (see Chapter 7).

TABLE 2.6

Reasons to reappraise the diagnosis

- No response to levodopa
- Early-onset severe bulbar disturbance (speech and swallowing)
- Early-onset balance problems
- Patient is wheelchair bound
- Lower-body parkinsonism
- Early-onset dementia
- Prominent eye-movement disorder
- Early-onset autonomic problems
  - bladder symptoms
  - sexual disturbance
  - postural hypotension

Imaging tests

Computed tomography (CT) or magnetic resonance imaging (MRI) scans are usually not needed for diagnosis, but a brain scan should be performed if parkinsonism is purely unilateral or otherwise atypical, or if additional signs (pyramidal) are present. CT or MRI may also be used to rule out a space-occupying lesion, vascular disease and normal-pressure hydrocephalus. This last condition causes lower-body parkinsonism, cognitive decline and early bladder symptoms.

Recently, the use of diffusion-weighted (MR) imaging (DWI) and diffusion tensor (MR) imaging (DTI) has been explored and developed in an effort to differentiate idiopathic Parkinson's disease from parkinsonism due to other causes such as MSA. DWI reflects a quantifiable coefficient known as the apparent diffusion coefficient (ADC), and preliminary reports suggest that idiopathic Parkinson's disease produces substantially higher regional ADC values than does MSA. DWI is also thought to differentiate between MSA and PSP. Further studies using this potentially widely available technique are under way.

Transcranial ultrasound scanning reveals characteristic hyperecho-genicity of the substantia nigra in patients with early Parkinson's disease. This indicates excessive iron deposition in the nigra, and some researchers have suggested the technique could be used as a screening tool for diagnosis of the disease. However, the technique needs to be validated in large-scale studies before widespread use can be advocated.

Single-photon emission computed tomography (SPECT) with DaTSCAN™. DaTSCAN™, an ethanolic solution containing a radioiodine-labeled cocaine derivative, is administered intravenously 3–6 hours before imaging by SPECT. The radiopharmaceutical binds with presynaptic dopamine transporters, enabling an assessment of neuronal degeneration to be made (Figure 2.3). SPECT can be used to confirm a positive clinical examination and also to differentiate difficult clinical cases in which essential tremor (which is likely to show a normal image) may mimic parkinsonian tremor (which shows an abnormal image). This type of imaging also apears to have a close correlation with the progression of Parkinson's disease. However, it is unable to differentiate between Parkinson's disease, MSA and PSP.

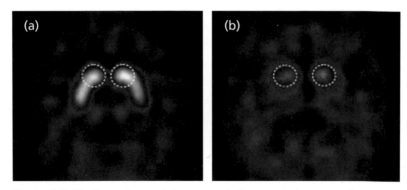

Figure 2.3 Single-photon emission computed tomography scans using DaTSCAN™, showing transverse images of the striatum and uptake of the radiopharmaceutical in dopamine-producing neurons. (a) Characteristic 'comma' shape and circular 'full stop' (as marked) in a normal brain, indicating uptake in the putamen and caudate, respectively. (b) Loss of uptake in the putamen due to Parkinson's disease, although uptake in the caudate (as marked by the circle) is initially preserved. Images courtesy of GE Healthcare.

Other tests. A positron emission tomography (PET) scan with fluorodopa can localize dopamine deficiency in the basal ganglia (see Figure 1.4), while autonomic tests and sphincter electromyography may support a diagnosis of MSA. PET, while more accurate than SPECT, is only available in research-based studies and is not routinely indicated in clinical practice.

Further investigations for young-onset or atypical disease include:

- measurement of copper and ceruloplasmin levels to rule out Wilson's disease
- tests to identify the gene for Huntington's disease
- tests to identify the gene for dentatorubral-pallidoluysian atrophy
- tests for spinocerebellar ataxia (particularly type 3), neuro-ferritinopathy and other neuronal brain-iron-accumulation syndromes
- syphilis serology
- measurement of manganese levels (see Welding-related parkinsonism, page 19).
- measurement of antibasal ganglia antibodies.

Referral

Current opinion and guidelines recommend that all patients with a 'suspected' diagnosis of Parkinson's disease must be referred untreated to a specialist who can reliably differentiate between Parkinson's disease and other parkinsonian syndromes. Ongoing care can be managed by the primary care team, but initiation of treatment in primary care is discouraged.

Differential diagnosis

Referral to a specialist is essential to ensure diagnosis is as accurate as possible (approximately 96% certainty in specialist centers). The key differential diagnoses include essential tremor, drug-induced parkinsonism, vascular pseudoparkinsonism and the Parkinson-plus syndromes such as MSA, PSP, dementia with Lewy bodies and corticobasal ganglionic degeneration (see Chapter 7 – Other parkinsonian syndromes).

Key points – diagnosis

- Most cases of Parkinson's disease are recognizable at an early stage, but can be misdiagnosed if tremor is absent.
- Characteristic motor symptoms include tremor, bradykinesia, a hurried shuffling gait, freezing episodes, rigidity and a bent posture.
- Non-motor symptoms include depression, dementia, sleep disorders, bowel and bladder problems, fatigue, apathy and pain; although common, these symptoms are often overlooked.
- There are no specific tests for the diagnosis of Parkinson's disease, but DaTSCAN™ with single-photon emission computed tomography is becoming widely available, and can help to support a clinical diagnosis.
- Patients with idiopathic Parkinson's disease show a significant and sustained response to dopaminergic agents.
- Brain imaging is not typically used to diagnose Parkinson's disease, but may help to rule out tumors, vascular disease and normal-pressure hydrocephalus; transcranial ultrasound scanning reveals characteristic hypoechogenicity of the substantia nigra.

Key references

Albanese A, Bonuccelli U, Brefel C et al. Consensus statement on the role of acute dopaminergic challenge in Parkinson's disease. *Mov Disord* 2001;16:197–201.

Chaudhuri KR, Healy DG, Schapira AH; National Institute for Health and Clinical Excellence. The non-motor symptoms of Parkinson's disease: diagnosis and management. *Lancet Neurol* 2006;5:235–45.

Chaudhuri KR, Martinez-Martin P, Schapira AH et al. International multicenter pilot study of the first comprehensive self-completed non-motor symptoms questionnaire for Parkinson's disease: the NMS Quest study. *Mov Disord* 2006;21:916–23.

Fahn S, Elton RL; members of the UPDRS Development Committee. Unified Parkinson's Disease Rating Scale. In: Fahn S, Marsden CD, Calne DB, Goldstein M, eds. *Recent Developments in Parkinson's Disease*, vol 2. Florham Park, NJ: Macmillan Health Care Information, 1987:153–63, 293–304. www.mdvu.org/pdf/updrs.pdf www.mdvu.org/pdf/upddf.pdf

Hoehn MM, Yahr MD. Parkinsonism: onset, progression, and mortality. *Neurology* 1998;50:318 (reprinted from *Neurology* 1967;17:427–42).

National Institute for Health and Clinical Excellence. *Parkinson's Disease. National Clinical Guideline for Diagnosis and Management in Primary and Secondary Care.* London: Royal College of Physicians, June 2006. http://guidance.nice.org. uk/CG35/guidance/pdf/English

Nutt JG, Wooten GF. Clinical practice. Diagnosis and initial management of Parkinson's disease. *N Engl J Med* 2005;353:1021–7.

Olanow CW, Watts RL, Koller WC. An algorithm (decision tree) for the management of Parkinson's disease (2001): treatment guidelines. *Neurology* 2001;56(11suppl5): S1–88.

Paviour DC, Thornton JS, Lees AJ, Jager HR. Diffusion-weighted magnetic resonance imaging differentiates Parkinsonian variant of multiple-system atrophy from progressive supranuclear palsy. *Mov Disord* 2007;22:68–74.

Piccini P, Brooks DJ. New developments of brain imaging for Parkinson's disease and related disorders. *Mov Disord* 2006;21: 2035–41.

Samii A, Nutt JG, Ransom BR. Parkinson's disease. *Lancet* 2004;363:1783–93.

History

In the 1920s, treatment of parkinsonism focused on the development of a vaccine that would prevent postencephalitic parkinsonism. Subsequently, pharmacological treatment has become the mainstay of management of Parkinson's disease. The first drugs, the belladonna alkaloids used in the 1860s, were replaced by the synthetic anticholinergic drugs benzhexol and benztropine in the 1940s. During the 1960s, Birkmayer and Hornykiewicz, Barbeau et al. and Cotzias et al. demonstrated the dramatic clinical effects of high-dose, oral levodopa therapy, revolutionizing the treatment of Parkinson's disease.

Levodopa is a precursor to dopamine and restores the dopamine lost due to degeneration of striatonigral cells. It has improved the quality of patients' lives substantially, and appears to have led to a reduction in mortality from three-times normal to near-normal life expectancy. Conversion of levodopa to dopamine occurs by dopa decarboxylation in the brain (Figure 3.1), and can also occur outside the blood–brain barrier, where it may lead to side effects such as nausea and postural hypotension. The addition of a peripheral decarboxylase inhibitor that does not cross the blood–brain barrier, such as carbidopa or benserazide, inhibits dopa decarboxylase in the rest of the body and reduces side effects. The bioavailability of levodopa has been enhanced further by the emergence of drugs such as tolcapone and entacapone, which inhibit catechol-O-methyl transferase (COMT), the enzyme principally responsible for the breakdown of dopamine.

When to initiate treatment

Precisely when to begin treatment is controversial (Table 3.1). Some experts advocate early treatment to provide maximum clinical benefit to patients, whereas others prefer to delay initiation of treatment in order to minimize the risk of levodopa-related motor complications.

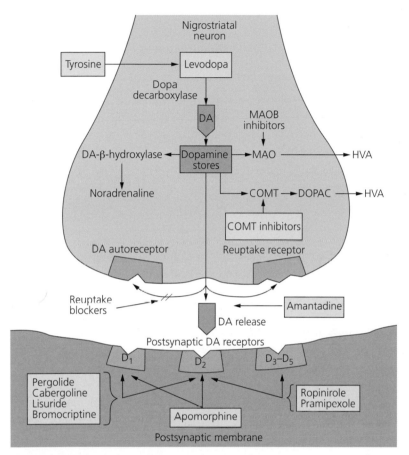

Figure 3.1 Dopamine metabolism and action of various dopaminergic drugs. COMT, catechol-*O*-methyl transferase; DA, dopamine; DOPAC, dihydroxy-phenylacetic acid; HVA, homovanillic acid; MAO, monoamine oxidase.

PDLIFE study. The argument for treatment of Parkinson's disease at diagnosis has been strengthened by the recent publication of the UK's prospective PDLIFE study, a national audit of the quality of life of people with Parkinson's disease. Findings indicate a progressive and significant deterioration in the self-reported health status of patients with Parkinson's disease who are left untreated at diagnosis compared with those who are treated. The work will reignite the debate of whether to initiate treatment of the disease at diagnosis or whether to adopt a 'wait and watch' policy, which is supported by the issue of

TABLE 3.1

Factors to consider when starting treatment

- Involvement of dominant hand relative to non-dominant hand
- Effect on employment/occupation
- The particular subtype of Parkinson's disease (bradykinesia-dominant disease may require earlier treatment than tremor-dominant disease)
- The individual sentiments of patients and carers (offer informed choice)

neuroprotection. Nevertheless, as Albin and Frey's critique demonstrates, the issue of neuroprotection in Parkinson's disease remains controversial.

Study results. Results of experiments with cultured dopaminergic neurons and with rats suggest that levodopa may be toxic to dopamine neurons; it is postulated that levodopa is converted to toxic dopamine metabolites that cause damage by the production of free radicals such as hydrogen peroxide. The substantia nigra is at risk because it contains high concentrations of catalysts, such as iron, for free-radical production, and low concentrations of free-radical scavengers. However, there is no firm evidence that levodopa is toxic to the human nigrostriatal pathway. A recent postmortem study of five patients with essential tremor, who were mistakenly given sustained levodopa therapy, found no evidence of damage to nigral cells; this should reassure many patients receiving long-term levodopa.

There is also concern that fluctuating levels of dopa may prime the brain for dyskinesia. The development of dyskinesias has been shown to adversely affect patients' and carers' quality of life, and to at least double the cost of care. Evidence for initiating treatment with a dopamine agonist comprises four published monotherapy trials comparing dopamine agonists (ropinirole, pramipexole, cabergoline and pergolide) with levodopa in previously untreated patients over a 4–5-year period.

Caution is necessary when comparing results, owing to methodological variability, but all the studies suggested that up to 50% fewer dyskinesias developed in those treated with a dopamine agonist rather than levodopa, which can be reserved for use when the effects of the dopamine agonist wear off.

Furthermore, preliminary evidence from positron emission tomography (PET) scans, comparing patients treated with ropinirole and pramipexole with those taking levodopa or being rescued by levodopa, suggests a slower annual rate of cell loss in patients treated with ropinirole and pramipexole.

The REAL-PET study (Ropinirole as EArly therapy versus Levodopa – PET study) showed that the loss of dopamine terminal function (a marker of progression of Parkinson's disease, measured by 18-fluorodopa uptake during PET scanning; see Figure 1.4) was significantly slower (approximately 30%; $p = 0.022$) in those taking ropinirole than in those receiving levodopa. Although motor scores were significantly better in patients receiving levodopa than those receiving ropinirole, treatment with ropinirole resulted in significantly fewer dyskinesias and possibly a significantly slower rate of progression of Parkinson's disease.

The CALM-PD study (Comparison of the Agonist pramipexole vs Levodopa on Motor complications in Parkinson's Disease study), in which dopamine transporter imaging was used as a surrogate marker for progression of Parkinson's disease, compared the response of patients taking the non-ergot dopamine agonist pramipexole with those taking levodopa. In patients initially treated with pramipexole, the rate of loss of striatal uptake of iodine-123-β-carbomethoxy-3β-4-iodophenyltropane (^{123}I-β-CIT) – a measure of presynaptic dopamine neuronal degeneration – was lower than in those taking levodopa during a 46-month period.

These results are similar to those observed in the REAL-PET study, and there is speculation among researchers regarding a neuroprotective role of ropinirole and pramipexole. This is a controversial notion, because the trial design does not take non-motor symptoms into account and cannot exclude the regulatory effect of drugs on the imaging findings.

The ELLDOPA study (Early versus Late LevoDOPA in Parkinson's disease study) more recently evaluated previously untreated patients with Parkinson's disease randomized to three doses (150, 300 or 600 mg) of levodopa or placebo. Levodopa-treated patients showed a significant improvement in motor scores at all three doses compared with those receiving placebo. Single-photon emission computed tomography (SPECT) imaging suggested an increased rate of decline of striatal ^{123}I-β-CIT uptake in the levodopa-treated arm compared with the placebo arm. This anomalous observation further deepens the confusion surrounding the use of imaging findings as surrogate markers, the link between imaging findings and clinical outcome, and whether in-vivo neuroprotection trials can really be performed.

The TEMPO study. More recently, the 'randomized delayed start' strategy has been adopted, such as that used in the TVP-1012 (rasagiline) as Early Monotherapy for Parkinson's disease Outpatients (TEMPO) study. Patients were randomized to either early or delayed treatment with rasagiline, a new, second-generation monoamine oxidase B (MAOB) inhibitor. Those who received delayed treatment had worse motor scores (assessed by the Unified Parkinson's Disease Rating Scale [UPDRS]) than those who were initiated on rasagiline. This strategy may suggest a possible neuroprotective effect of rasagiline and, if clinically proven, would reinforce a policy shift in favor of early treatment of Parkinson's disease rather than symptom-led delayed treatment.

Current guidelines. On the basis of these findings, the initial use of dopamine agonists or other levodopa-sparing agents such as rasagiline, oral selegiline or amantadine, to delay the start of levodopa therapy, has been advocated.

However, the guidelines of the UK's National Institute for Health and Clinical Excellence (NICE), issued in June 2006 (page 63), and the American Academy of Neurology (AAN) 2006 guideline for the management of Parkinson's disease suggest that there is insufficient evidence to support the use of dopamine agonists over levodopa, and recommend initial treatment with levodopa preparations, dopamine agonists or MAOB inhibitors. The greater gain in motor function with levodopa is offset by the significantly lower risk of dyskinesias with dopamine agonists.

The guidelines issued by the European Federation of Neurological Societies (EFNS) in 2006 differ somewhat. The EFNS recommends initial treatment with MAOB inhibitors, amantadine or an anticholinergic (from level B evidence), levodopa and orally active non-ergot dopamine agonists. In the UK, however, use of anticholinergics as an initial treatment is not recommended owing to a possible risk of worsening cognitive function. In later and more advanced disease, adjunctive treatment with dopamine agonists, subcutaneous apomorphine therapy and deep brain surgery (stimulation of the subthalamic nucleus being the preferred option) are recommended. At all stages, multidisciplinary care and management of non-motor symptoms are recommended.

In practice, all patients should be helped to make an informed choice. Many younger patients will choose a levodopa-sparing strategy, while older patients may prefer levodopa therapy.

Levodopa

Patients with typical Parkinson's disease respond to levodopa almost immediately, although in some cases a delayed effect is seen after prolonged treatment. The beneficial response to levodopa can often be assessed after a single test dose (see Table 2.5).

However, there may be significant false-positive results, given that patients with multiple-system atrophy or progressive supranuclear palsy may also respond to levodopa initially. In addition, the test does not allow for the delayed positive 'long-duration' effect of levodopa. In resistant cases, the maximum tolerated dose (up to 2 g/day) should be tried for at least 1 month before the patient is declared unresponsive.

Levodopa therapy should be started at the minimal effective dose (usually 50–100 mg/day), in combination with a decarboxylase inhibitor given three times daily. Side effects, such as light-headedness or nausea, may be relieved by taking the medication with food or by increasing the dose of decarboxylase inhibitor. Side effects usually settle but, if persistent, can be prevented by using a peripheral dopamine antagonist, such as domperidone, 20 mg three times daily. Some complications may, however, persist in the long term (Table 3.2).

TABLE 3.2

Levodopa-related complications

Short term

Gastrointestinal	• Nausea, vomiting, gastritis
Cardiovascular	• Postural hypotension

Long term

Motor

Fluctuations	• 'Wearing-off' phenomenon (end-of-dose deterioration)
	• Random 'on/off' oscillations
	• Delayed 'on' response
	• Drug-resistant 'off' phenomenon (dose failure)
	• Early-morning akinesia
	• Freezing
	• Diphasic dyskinesia
Dyskinesia	• Peak-dose choreic turning 'on'
Non-motor	• Pain, akathisia, restless legs
('off' period related)	• Sweating, tachycardia, dyspnea
	• Depression, panic attacks, hyperventilation, screaming
	• 'Off' period dystonia
Neuropsychiatric	• Hallucinations
	• Delirium and paranoid psychosis
	• Hypersexuality
Sleep related	• Nightmares/vivid dreams
	• Fragmented sleep

Levodopa formulations

Controlled-release preparations of levodopa, 200 mg or 100 mg, have no significant advantages over immediate-release preparations apart from their use in treating nocturnal disabilities. Such preparations have reduced

bioavailability, and many patients dislike the longer lead time before improvement. Combining controlled-release and shorter-acting preparations is not advisable because the effect is difficult to predict.

Addition of a catechol-O-methyl transferase (COMT) inhibitor, entacapone, to the traditional combination of levodopa and a decarboxylase inhibitor (carbidopa) is now licensed for the treatment of later-stage Parkinson's disease that is no longer stabilized on a levodopa/decarboxylase preparation. Studies to establish the role of this new formulation as initiation therapy for Parkinson's disease are under way.

Intraduodenal/jejunal infusion of levodopa offers an alternative route of administration in very advanced Parkinson's disease when other treatments have failed, and in patients not suitable for deep brain stimulation (see pages 71–4) or apomorphine (see pages 53–4). Using a portable infusion pump the enteral gel is delivered continuously through a percutaneous endoscopic gastrostomy tube into the duodenum, where it is absorbed and produces a steady plasma level. Studies have shown that this infusion is effective in controlling motor fluctuations in advanced Parkinson's disease and reduces dyskinesias. It also enables the patient to discontinue oral dopaminergic treatment and apomorphine infusion. It is licensed in several countries as an 'orphan' drug.

Dopamine agonists

Dopamine agonists stimulate dopamine receptors directly and so bypass the degenerating presynaptic nigrostriatal neurons. Five types of dopamine receptors (D_1–D_5) have been identified so far; these are broadly divided into:

- D_1-like receptors (D_1 and D_5) – linked to adenylate cyclase
- D_2-like receptors (D_2, D_3 and D_4) – not linked to adenylate cyclase.

Improvement in motor function is generally attributed to D_1 and D_2 receptors, which are densely concentrated in the striatum (caudate nucleus and putamen). D_3 receptors are localized in the limbic regions that are important for regulation of behavior, mood and emotion. Ease of use, side effects and relative cost determine which dopamine agonist to choose (Tables 3.3 and 3.4).

TABLE 3.3

Dopamine agonists

Agonist*	Receptor selectivity	Typical dose (mg/day)[†]	Indications and advantages
Ergot			
Bromocriptine	D_1- D_2++	5–20 (1.25–30)	Adjunctive[‡] Inexpensive
Lisuride	D_1++ D_2++++	1–3 (0.6–5)	Adjunctive[‡] Subcutaneous route possible
Pergolide	D_1++ D_2++++ D_3++	1–3 (0.75–5)	Adjunctive[‡]
Cabergoline	D_1++ D_2++++	2–4 (1–12)	Adjunctive[‡] or monotherapy Once-daily dosing
Non-ergot			
Ropinirole	D_2+++ D_3++++	3–18 (1–24)[¶]	Adjunctive[‡] or monotherapy
Pramipexole	D_2++++ D_3++++	1.5–4.5 (0.75–6)	Adjunctive[‡] or monotherapy
Rotigotine	D_1++ D_2++ D_3++++	4–8[††] (2–16)	Adjunctive or monotherapy
Subcutaneous			
Apomorphine	D_1++++ D_2++++ D_3+	10–80 (3–120)	Adjunctive[‡]

*Preferably, all agonists should be used after pretreatment with domperidone, 20 mg three times daily, with the possible exception of cabergoline. Somnolence may occur with the use of all dopamine agonists, particularly in older patients (> 75 years) and at high doses. Recently, there has been increasing concern about dopamine dysregulation syndrome (compulsive gambling associated with dopaminergic treatment in individuals with a history of gambling, substance addiction and young-onset Parkinson's disease; see page 55).
[†]Values in parentheses indicate dose ranges used occasionally in clinical practice. Common dose ranges are presented without parentheses.
[‡]In advanced Parkinson's disease.

Additional uses	Side effects, established/probable
RLS	Fibrosis, ankle edema, hypersexuality, ergot side effects (Table 3.4) Neuropsychiatric side effects (particularly hallucinations)
RLS; nocturia	Ergot side effects, cardiac valve fibrosis,[§] ankle edema, hypersexuality
RLS; nighttime symptoms; early-morning dystonia	Ergot side effects, cardiac valve fibrosis,[§] ankle edema, hypersexuality
RLS; tremor**	Somnolence, neuropsychiatric side effects
RLS; tremor;** depression	Somnolence, insomnia, neuropsychiatric side effects
Nighttime symptoms; skin irritation; postural hypotension	Nausea/vomiting
RLS; dyskinesias; pain ('off' period); dystonia; impotence	Skin nodules, postural hypotension, nausea/vomiting, substance abuse (homeostatic hedonistic dysregulation)

[§]Occasional cases reported; pleuropulmonary and retroperitoneal fibrosis are serious ergot-related side effects, and patients treated with these drugs should be monitored carefully every 6 or 12 months with measurement of erythrocyte sedimentation rate, renal function test, chest X-ray or CT scanning and lung function test if indicated.
[¶]Ropinirole monotherapy can be initiated with a starter and continuation pack that titrates the dose up to 9 mg/day, thus avoiding underdosing.
**Beneficial effect suggested by open studies and anecdotal evidence but not confirmed in controlled studies.
[††]Maximum dose for monotherapy.
–, antagonist action at receptor; +, agonist action at receptor; RLS, restless legs syndrome.

TABLE 3.4

Ergot side effects

Common
- Nausea and/or vomiting
- Neuropsychiatric effects, e.g. hallucinations
- Postural hypotension

Side effects requiring regular monitoring
- Fibrosis (cardiac, retroperitoneal or pulmonary)

Rare
- Erythromelalgia or vasospasm
- Aggravation of peripheral circulatory failure
- Priapism

Comparative studies of the efficacy of the newer dopamine agonists are scarce. Two studies (one double-blind, one open) comparing pergolide with cabergoline (the longest-acting dopamine agonist) indicated that cabergoline may have superior efficacy over pergolide, particularly in relation to the treatment of nighttime disabilities, such as nocturnal freezing, 'off' periods, early-morning dystonia, pain and restless legs syndrome. Previous studies have compared bromocriptine with ropinirole.

However, there is increasing concern regarding the use of pergolide and cabergoline because of studies showing an association with ergot-related cardiac valvular disease. Pergolide is now only recommended after pretreatment echocardiography (ECG), with regular monitoring by ECG during treatment. Likewise, before cabergoline is started patients must have a chest X-ray and renal function test, and erythrocyte sedimentation rate (ESR) should be measured. Their lung and cardiac function should also be regularly monitored.

In this respect, non-ergot dopamine agonists such as pramipexole, ropinirole and the rotigotine skin patch are preferable. Longer-acting agonists such as the rotigotine skin patch and once-daily ropinirole (not yet released) may also be used to exploit the long half-life of these drugs to attempt continuous dopaminergic stimulation (CDS) in real life.

The longer half-life of some dopamine agonists, and also their receptor specificity, may help in the provision of a more sustained and selective motor effect with fewer side effects (Table 3.5). CDS is a relatively modern concept that has been shown to reduce the severity and incidence of dyskinesias based on the fact that pulsatile delivery of dopamine to the deafferented dopamine receptors in the striatum is likely to be dyskinesogenic. CDS may prevent or reverse motor complications because it does not prime the basal ganglia for involuntary movements as much as agents that produce pulsatile stimulation. CDS may also improve some aspects of sleep in patients with Parkinson's disease. However, Nutt recently reinforced the idea that CDS remains a theoretical concept, and the effect of CDS on dyskinesias, to date, has never been tested in a robust randomized clinical trial.

TABLE 3.5

Comparison of elimination half-life of dopamine agonists and levodopa

Drug	Elimination half-life (hours)	Dosing regimen
Bromocriptine	6	t.d.s.
Pergolide	7–16	t.d.s.
Pramipexole	8–12	t.d.s.
Ropinirole	6	t.d.s.
Cabergoline	63–68	o.d.
Rotigotine	5–7	o.d
Lisuride	2–4	b.d. or t.d.s.
Apomorphine	0.5	s.c. 12–24 h/day
Levodopa (immediate release)	1	b.d. or t.d.s.
Levodopa (controlled release)	1.5–2	o.d. or b.d.

o.d., once daily; b.d., twice daily; t.d.s., three times daily; s.c. subcutaneous.

In practice, dopamine agonists are also useful for smoothing the 'on/off' fluctuations secondary to levodopa, as well as the many theoretical advantages listed in Table 3.6.

Ropinirole and pramipexole are well-established non-ergot dopamine agonists in widespread clinical use in early and advanced Parkinson's disease. Both are effective in early and late disease as monotherapy and adjunctive therapy. Pramipexole, in particular, has been investigated for antidepressant and antianxiety effects, and a recent parallel-group randomized study in people with Parkinson's disease has indicated that pramipexole has antidepressant effects comparable to sertraline.

In the 1990s, a controversial paper reported that eight patients who had taken either pramipexole or ropinirole fell asleep while driving, causing accidents. In Europe, this led to a driving ban for patients taking either of the two drugs, although the ban has now been lifted. Since then, similar episodes of unintended sleep have been reported in patients taking other dopaminergic drugs. Daytime sleepiness is likely to be a part of the disease process, which could be aggravated by the use of dopaminergic drugs. This important side effect is discussed in greater detail below (see Sleep disorders).

TABLE 3.6

Theoretical advantages of dopamine agonists

- Direct stimulation of dopamine receptors, bypassing degenerating nigrostriatal neurons
- Potential for selective dopamine receptor (D_1, D_2 or D_3) activation
- Longer striatal half-life compared with levodopa
- No intermediate step requiring enzymatic conversion to active drug
- No competition with larger neutral amino-acid transport in gut or at blood–brain barrier
- Controversial clinical evidence for possible neuroprotective disease-modifying effects
- Delayed appearance of levodopa-related side effects

Rotigotine is the first transdermally delivered non-ergot dopamine agonist shown to be effective in early and advanced Parkinson's disease. Unlike the other non-ergot dopamine agonists it is effective in a once-daily application, and provides a theoretically attractive option for CDS by achieving constant plasma levels over 24 hours. In parkinsonian primate and mouse models, treatment with rotigotine produces virtually no dyskinesias.

In addition to D_3 activity, rotigotine also has considerable affinity for the D_1 receptor, unlike the other non-ergot dopamine agonists pramipexole and ropinirole. This is theoretically important because D_1 activity is thought to synergistically enhance the effect mediated via D_2-like receptors. Rotigotine appears to have no affinity for $5\text{-}HT_{2b}$ receptors, which have been implicated in the pathogenesis of fibrotic side effects associated with ergot dopamine agonists, particularly cardiac valvulopathy.

Transdermal delivery also offers the advantage of preventing interaction with food and the first-pass metabolism associated with oral drugs. Approximately 1200 patients were enrolled worldwide in phase 3 trials in which rotigotine provided effective relief from the symptoms of both early and advanced Parkinson's disease.

In clinical trials, a rotigotine patch was associated with a reaction at the site of application in 39–44% of patients, although only a small subset had a severe reaction. The risk is reduced by changing the application site on a daily basis.

Apomorphine is a highly potent D_1 and D_2 agonist that also acts on D_3 receptors but has no opioid properties. It has a short half-life and is usually administered subcutaneously, either as a 'rescue' injection or by an infusion pump over 12, 18 or 24 hours. The effect of oral or rectal apomorphine is less reliable; delivery by transdermal iontophoresis, or a buccal, intranasal or rectal route is under investigation. Occasionally, patients can stop taking levodopa, but most need regular doses in addition to apomorphine.

Apomorphine infusion benefits patients with refractory motor response fluctuations and diphasic dyskinesias. Continuous subcutaneous administration may be very useful in the later stages of

53

the disease, producing a continuous antidyskinetic effect and smoothing 'on/off' fluctuations. In the case of injections, a response occurs after 10–15 minutes and lasts for 45–60 minutes. Self-injection, in a manner similar to the self-injection of insulin by diabetics, is ideal for 'rescuing' patients from disabling 'off' periods. The treatment is labor-intensive and requires specialist nursing care. In the UK, 'shared care' guidelines have been developed to help the delivery of apomorphine therapy, clearly setting out the shared responsibilities of primary and secondary care providers. Daily rotation of injection sites may prevent skin nodules, while local ultrasound therapy and skin massage can help to treat existing nodules.

Domperidone (not available in the USA), 20 mg three times daily for at least 2 weeks, is recommended for use with all dopamine agonists, and is compulsory with apomorphine to prevent severe nausea and vomiting. However, domperidone can often be stopped after several months of dopaminergic therapy. In the USA, trimethobenzamide, 250 mg three times daily, is used in conjunction with apomorphine to prevent nausea.

Sleep disorders. Unintended or abnormal sleepiness is a potentially dangerous adverse effect in patients taking dopaminergic agents. As well as the incidents reported in patients taking ropinirole and pramipexole (see above), similar episodes have been reported in patients taking pergolide, bromocriptine, cabergoline, apomorphine and levodopa. However, abnormal sleepiness has also been described in patients with Parkinson's disease at the time of diagnosis, when they are not yet receiving any dopamine-replacement therapy. Daytime sleepiness is, therefore, likely to be a combined effect of the disease process and dopaminergic drug treatment, and not a novel event related solely to the use of dopamine agonists.

A small percentage of patients with Parkinson's disease (possibly 0.5–1%) with excessive daytime sleepiness, may exhibit sudden onset of sleep resembling narcolepsy. For this reason, older patients receiving dopaminergic therapy should be assessed using both the Epworth Sleepiness Scale (for excessive daytime sleepiness) and the Parkinson's Disease Sleep Scale (PDSS). A pragmatic view is that those who score more than 10 out of 24 on the Epworth scale, or less than 5 on item 15 of the PDSS, should be advised to exercise caution when driving, or preferably not to drive at all during the titration phase of therapy.

Studies suggest that somnolence is at its worst when dopaminergic therapy, particularly treatment with dopamine agonists, is being initiated and titrated up. In 'sleepy' patients, polysomnography may identify a subset of people with a phenotype similar to that for narcolepsy, or it may unearth sleep apnea as a cause of daytime sleepiness.

Dopamine dysregulation syndrome, which resembles addiction, has recently been described in mostly young male patients with Parkinson's disease. The patients exhibit complex neuropsychiatric symptoms, including wandering, compulsive gambling, punding (repetitive, meaningless behavior), drug hoarding and hypersexuality. They may also be addicted to oral dopamine agonists, levodopa or apomorphine. Compulsive behaviors may include compulsive shopping, night eating, addiction to computers and 'hobbyisms'. As well as dopamine dysregulation syndrome, the condition has been variously known as:

- homeostatic hedonistic dysregulation
- impulse dysregulation
- compulsive behavior syndrome
- reward-seeking behavior.

Men with early-onset Parkinson's disease and a history of alcohol misuse, illicit drug use or affective disorders may be susceptible to this syndrome. Abnormal dopamine release in the nucleus accumbens in response to a reward has been postulated as a possible mechanism. The treatment is complex and requires slow withdrawal of dopamine agonists, use of atypical neuroleptics and/or antidepressants, counseling and input from a neuropsychiatrist.

Fibrosis. The risk of serosal fibrosis in relation to ergot-derived drugs was first described in 1966. Recently, there have been several reports of cardiac, retroperitoneal and pleuropulmonary fibrosis in patients taking ergot-derived dopamine agonists such as pergolide, cabergoline and bromocriptine. Serosal fibrosis is a serious complication that is often irreversible.

Pergolide, in particular, has been associated with cardiac valve fibrosis and regurgitation. All patients taking pergolide should have annual echocardiography and renal function tests, measurement of ESR and a chest X-ray. Those using other ergot-derived dopamine agonists such as cabergoline must have baseline renal function tests, ESR measurement and a chest X-ray before treatment is started. The increased affinity of ergot-derived dopamine agonists for 5-HT$_{2b}$ receptors has been cited as a possible mechanism.

Catechol-*O*-methyl transferase inhibitors

COMT metabolizes dopamine and levodopa, producing two inactive metabolites, 3-O-methyl-dopamine and 3-O-methyl-dopa. Two COMT inhibitors, tolcapone and entacapone, are available; they extend the plasma half-life of levodopa, thus increasing the concentrations of levodopa and dopamine within the brain (Table 3.7; Figure 3.2). COMT inhibition prolongs 'on' time by 30–60%, which may increase the duration of, but not worsen, peak-dose dyskinesias.

Tolcapone blocks COMT in both the peripheral and central nervous systems. In November 1998, the European Medical Evaluation Agency withdrew tolcapone in the EU because of three cases of fatal fulminant hepatitis; sales were also suspended in Canada and Australia. In the USA, the Food and Drug Administration (FDA) recommended that

TABLE 3.7

Catechol-*O*-methyl transferase inhibitors in Parkinson's disease

- *Never* use entacapone without levodopa
- Tolcapone should be used with regular liver function tests only
- Useful for early or moderately advanced disease with motor fluctuations and 'wearing off'
- Reduce levodopa dose by about 20% in dyskinetic patients, as use may worsen diphasic dyskinesia
- Entacapone and tolcapone may color urine reddish-orange
- Sudden withdrawal may cause an akinetic crisis

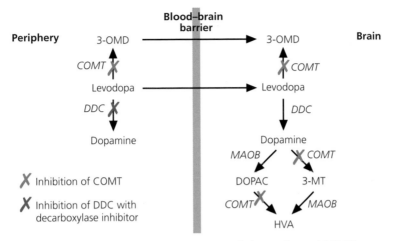

Figure 3.2 The mechanism of catechol-O-methyl transferase (COMT) inhibition. DDC, dopa decarboxylase; DOPAC, dihydroxyphenylacetic acid; HVA, homovanillic acid; MAOB, monoamine oxidase B; 3-MT, 3-methoxy-tyramine; 3-OMD, 3-O-methyl-dopa.

regular liver function tests be performed. Tolcapone has now been re-released in Europe, but its use must be accompanied by regular blood tests to monitor liver function. The FDA now advises that levels of alanine and aspartate transaminase (ALT/AST) should be determined at baseline, then every 2–4 weeks during the first 6 months of therapy and then at intervals deemed clinically relevant. In the USA, tolcapone should be discontinued if ALT or AST levels exceed two times the normal upper limit. The patient consent form has been replaced with a patient acknowledgment form. The usual starting dose is 100 mg/day, increased to 200 mg three times daily. Dyskinesia and nausea are common side effects, but diarrhea is the most common reason for drug withdrawal. Patients should be warned that the drug may color their urine.

Entacapone, 200 mg with each dose of levodopa, acts only peripherally, unlike tolcapone. No hepatobiliary side effects have been reported, and routine liver function tests are not required. The incidence of diarrhea is also less frequent than with tolcapone. Other side effects include hypotension, sedation, headache and dyskinesias. Patients should be forewarned that the drug may turn urine a reddish-orange color.

A combined formulation of entacapone, decarboxylase inhibitor and levodopa has recently been licensed for use in the USA, Europe and certain parts of Asia; the drug should make compliance easier for patients taking entacapone and is likely to be administered for treatment of early 'wearing-off' symptoms. Its use may be refined with a new scale/questionnaire designed to assess 'wearing off', as described by Stacy et al.

Monoamine oxidase B inhibitors

Selegiline, 10 mg once daily or 5 mg twice daily orally (or 1.25 mg once daily by buccal administration), is a selective, irreversible blocker of intra- and extraneuronal MAOB, and reduces metabolism of dopamine (Figure 3.3). The sublingual form of selegiline (1.25–2.5 mg/day) can be administered as an adjunct to levodopa in patients with fluctuations.

In animal models, selegiline blocks the conversion of MPTP to MPP+, which is toxic to dopaminergic neurons (see Figure 1.3). On this

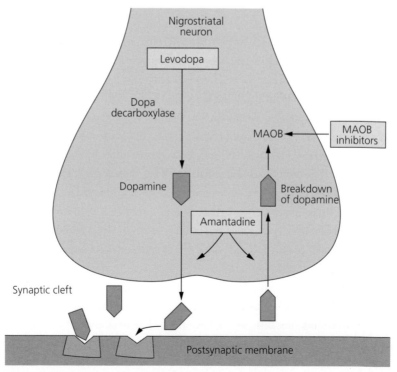

Figure 3.3 Action of presynaptic drugs.

basis, it was thought that MAOB inhibition with selegiline might slow the decline in human Parkinson's disease by neuroprotection. However, the double-blind, prospective, placebo-controlled DATATOP study (Deprenyl And Tocopherol Antioxidant Therapy for Parkinsonism study) in 1993, failed to confirm the neuroprotective property of selegiline. Furthermore, in the mid-1990s a report by the Parkinson's Disease Research Group (UK) suggested a 60% increase in mortality among patients receiving continued selegiline therapy, although this has not been substantiated.

The side effects of MAOB inhibition include hallucinations, sleep disorders, agitation, postural hypotension and withdrawal problems. Although a new formulation of selegiline is now available at a lower dose of 2.5 mg, which has a better safety profile, its clinical role remains unclear: it is not neuroprotective, and safety in older patients is uncertain. However, it can have a useful dopa-sparing effect and may stimulate drowsy patients.

Rasagiline is a new second-generation, irreversible, selective MAOB inhibitor that is administered orally at a dosage of 0.5–1 mg once daily. Approved dosing of this drug varies in different countries: the approved dose in Europe is 1 mg, while both 0.5 mg and 1 mg doses are approved in the USA, so that adjunctive therapy initiated at 0.5 mg can be raised to 1 mg if efficacy is insufficient at the lower dose. It is approximately five times more potent than selegiline, and, in animal models, rasagiline increased cellular antioxidant activity and antiapoptotic factors.

In clinical trials, patients started late on rasagiline appeared to have worse motor scores than those initiated on rasagiline, prompting some researchers to suggest that rasagiline may have a disease-modifying role in Parkinson's disease. Further research is required to confirm this hypothesis: the Attenuation of Disease progression with Azilect® Given Once-daily (ADAGIO) trial is under way at 129 centers in 14 countries to determine if treatment with once-daily rasagiline can modify the progression of Parkinson's disease.

Several randomized, controlled, clinical trials have shown rasagiline's efficacy as monotherapy or as an adjunct to levodopa in patients with Parkinson's disease.

Anticholinergics

Anticholinergics block the action of acetylcholine against dopamine within the basal ganglia (Figure 3.4). Data on the comparative efficacy of the different anticholinergic drugs are not available.

Commonly prescribed anticholinergics are benzhexol, benztropine, procyclidine, orphenadrine and biperiden (Table 3.8). These drugs may be a useful adjunct to levodopa therapy, helping to control rest-tremor and dystonia. They should be used with caution in older parkinsonian patients because of the risk of inducing a confusional state and aggravating dementia.

Side effects include urinary retention, constipation, blurred vision, precipitation of narrow-angle glaucoma, dry mouth, memory problems and confusion. If neuropsychiatric side effects necessitate withdrawal of anticholinergic therapy, this should be carried out slowly in order to avoid a withdrawal syndrome that itself includes a confusional state associated with akinesia and disorientation.

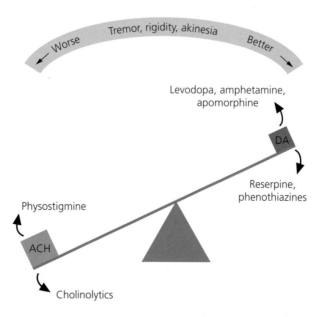

Figure 3.4 Dopamine–acetylcholine imbalance in Parkinson's disease. ACH, acetylcholine; DA, dopamine.

TABLE 3.8

Commonly prescribed anticholinergic drugs

Drug	Dosing regimen
Benzhexol in three divided doses	1 mg starting dose, increased to 6–8 mg daily
Benztropine in divided doses	0.5–1 mg starting dose, increased to 4–6 mg daily (can be given intramuscularly in a crisis)
Procyclidine	2–5 mg t.d.s. after meals
Orphenadrine	50 mg intramuscularly t.d.s.
Biperiden hydrochloride	2 mg daily

t.d.s., three times daily.

Other drugs

Amantadine, 100–400 mg daily, is an antiviral agent with an antiparkinsonian effect. Its mechanisms of action include:

- increased dopamine synthesis
- an amphetamine-like action releasing catecholamines from presynaptic stores
- blocking dopamine and noradrenaline reuptake
- mild anticholinergic action
- antiglutamate action by antagonism at the N-methyl-D-aspartate receptors.

The antiparkinsonian effect of amantadine is mild, and is useful in young patients to delay the introduction of levodopa. The effect is long-lasting, and patients may deteriorate markedly if the drug is withdrawn.

Amantadine should be given as a single dose in the morning to prevent sleep problems.

At high doses, amantadine has an anti-dyskinetic action that may last up to 9 months, but high doses can cause visual hallucinations, confusion and agitation. Amantadine can cause a specific discoloration of the legs called livedo reticularis.

Choice of treatment

All patients with Parkinson's disease who require drug treatment should be given the opportunity to make an informed choice from the range of treatment options available, including dopamine agonists, other levodopa-sparing agents, levodopa and combination therapy. Treatment should be based on the degree of disability, occupational needs, age, patient/clinician preferences and compliance issues.

In younger patients, the issue of neuroprotection and dyskinesias should be considered. Results of four controlled dopamine-agonist monotherapy trials have been published and suggest that initiation of treatment with an agonist is beneficial in the early stages of Parkinson's disease (see pages 43–4).

If levodopa is used and the dose is titrated to the response, most patients initially need 50–100 mg three times daily to produce a consistent effect without fluctuations. Within 2–3 years, most will need a more frequent dosage to avoid fluctuations; smaller, more frequent doses (every 2–3 hours) often lead to an overall increase in dose. COMT inhibitors or dopamine agonists can, however, be introduced instead of increasing the frequency of levodopa.

The main aims are to:
- keep the drug regimen as simple as possible
- aid compliance
- reduce the likelihood of side effects.

Theoretically, attempts should be made to stick to a regimen that mimics CDS as much as possible. Long-acting agents, or continuous delivery systems such as the rotigotine transdermal patch, or controlled-release preparations of other non-ergot dopamine agonists may be particularly useful in this regard.

Monitoring. Scales for monitoring Parkinson's disease, and thus the response to treatment, include:
- Unified Parkinson's Disease Rating Scale, which is currently being modified and validated by the Movement Disorder Society
- Hoehn and Yahr Disease Staging Scale (Table 3.9)
- Parkinson's Disease Questionnaire (long form – PDQ 39; short form – PDQ 8)

TABLE 3.9

The Hoehn and Yahr classification of Parkinson's disease

Stage	Characteristics
0	• No signs of disease
1	• Unilateral involvement only; minimal or no functional impairment
1.5	• Unilateral disease, plus axial involvement
2	• Bilateral disease, without impairment of balance
2.5	• Mild bilateral disease with recovery on pull test
3	• Mild to moderate bilateral disease; some postural instability; physically independent
4	• Severe disability; still able to walk or stand unassisted
5	• Wheelchair bound or bedridden unless aided

- EuroQol (patient-related quality of life)
- Carer Strain Index
- Epworth Sleepiness Scale
- Parkinson's Disease Sleep Scale
- Non-Motor Symptoms Questionnaire (NMSQuest; see Table 2.4)
- Non-Motor Symptoms Scale (NMSS).

Guidelines for the management of Parkinson's disease published in the UK by the NICE in June 2006 offer evidence-based advice issued by a multidisciplinary panel. Key recommendations are that patients and their carers should be involved in deciding their treatment and care, and that the choice of treatment should suit the patient's needs and preferences.

The following key points were identified as priorities for implementation.

- Any patient with a suspected diagnosis of Parkinson's disease should be seen by a specialist within 6 weeks after referral by the primary care physician. A specialist is defined as an individual with expertise in the differential diagnosis of Parkinson's disease.

Key points – drug treatment

- Levodopa restores the dopamine lost due to degeneration of striatonigral cells; patients with typical Parkinson's disease respond to levodopa almost immediately.
- Dopamine agonists are useful for smoothing the 'on/off' fluctuations secondary to levodopa therapy; some, such as rotigotine, may offer continuous dopaminergic stimulation in practice.
- Treatment decisions should be based on the degree of disability, occupational needs, age, patient/clinician preference and compliance issues; neuroprotection remains a theoretical argument, while dyskinesias are an important consideration in younger patients.
- Trial data indicate that treatment of Parkinson's disease could be initiated with levodopa, oral dopamine agonists or a monoamine oxidase B inhibitor.
- The findings of the PDLIFE study suggest that early initiation of treatment may be beneficial in terms of health-related quality of life.
- Daytime sleepiness is a part of the disease process that could be aggravated by the use of dopaminergic drugs; other potential problems include cardiac valve fibrosis with ergot dopamine agonists and compulsive behavioral syndromes with dopaminergic therapies.
- The treatment of non-motor symptoms is also important at all stages of Parkinson's disease.

- The diagnosis of Parkinson's disease should be reviewed every 6–12 months. The apomorphine and levodopa challenge tests should not be used to differentiate Parkinson's disease from atypical parkinsonian syndromes.
- Regular access to specialist nursing care, physiotherapy, occupational therapy and speech and language therapy should be available to patients.

- Patients and their carers should be given an opportunity to discuss palliative care issues.

No specific agents could be identified as the treatment of choice in either early or advanced disease. The guidelines also emphasise the need for considering non-motor symptoms at all stages of Parkinson's disease.

Guidelines for the management of Parkinson's disease in other countries are broadly similar to the NICE guidelines. They include those of the AAN, published in 2002 and modified in 2006, and those issued by the joint task force of the EFNS and the Movement Disorder Society's European Section in 2006.

Key references

Albin RL, Frey KA. Initial agonist treatment of Parkinson's disease: a critique. *Neurology* 2003;60:390–4.

Barbeau A, Sourkes TL, Murphy GF. J Ajuriaguerra (ed). Les catecholamines dans la maladie de Parkinson. In: *Monoamines et système nerveux central.* Paris: Masson, 1962:247–62.

Birkmayer W, Hornykiewicz O. Der l-Dioxyphenylalanin (= DOPA) Effekt beim Parkinson-Syndrom des Menschen: Zur Pathogenese und Behandlung der Parkinson-Akinese. *Arch Psychiatr Nervenkr* 1962;203: 560–74.

Chaudhuri KR, Pal S, Brefel-Courbon C. 'Sleep attacks' or 'unintended sleep episodes' occur with dopamine agonists: is this a class effect? *Drug Saf* 2002;25: 473–83.

Cotzias GC, Van Woert MH, Schiffer LM. Aromatic amino acids and modification of parkinsonism. *N Engl J Med* 1967;276:374–9.

Dhawan V, Healy DG, Pal S, Chaudhuri KR. Sleep-related problems of Parkinson's disease. *Age Ageing* 2006;35:220–8.

Grosset D, Taurah L, Burn DJ et al. A multicentre longitudinal observational study of changes in quality of life in people with Parkinson's disease left untreated at diagnosis. *J Neurol Neurosurg Psychiatry* 2007; in press (*JNNP Online*, 10 November 2006).

Horstink M, Tolosa E, Bonuccelli G et al. Review of the therapeutic management of Parkinson's disease. Report of a joint task force of the EFNS and the MDS-ES. Part I: early (uncomplicated) Parkinson's disease – Guideline 51. *Eur J Neurol* 2006; 13:1170–85.

Horstink M, Tolosa E, Bonuccelli G et al. Review of the therapeutic management of Parkinson's disease. Report of a joint task force of the EFNS and the MDS-ES. Part II: late (complicated) Parkinson's disease – Guideline 52. *Eur J Neurol* 2006; 13:1186–202.

LeWitt P. Rotigotine: a viewpoint by Peter LeWitt. *CNS Drugs* 2005;19:983–4.

Naidu Y, Chaudhuri KR. Transdermal rotigotine: a new non-ergot dopamine agonist for the treatment of Parkinson's disease. *Expert Opin Drug Deliv* 2007;4: 111–18.

National Institute for Health and Clinical Excellence. *Parkinson's Disease. Clinical Guidelines for Diagnosis and Management in Primary and Secondary Care.* London: Royal College of Physicians, June 2006. http://guidance.nice.org.uk/CG35/guidance/pdf/English

Nutt JG. Continuous dopaminergic stimulation: is it the answer to the motor complications of levodopa? *Mov Disord* 2007;22:1–9.

Nyholm D, Askmark H, Gomes-Trolin C et al. Optimising levodopa pharmacokinetics: intestinal infusion versus oral sustained-release tablets. *Clin Neuropharmacol* 2003;26: 156–63.

Olanow CW, Watts RL, Koller WC. An algorithm (decision tree) for the management of Parkinson's disease (2001): treatment guidelines. *Neurology* 2001;56(11suppl5): S1–88.

Olanow W, Schapira AH, Rascol O. Continuous dopamine-receptor stimulation in early Parkinson's disease. *Trends Neurosci* 2000;23: S117–26.

Parkinson Study Group. A controlled trial of rasagiline in early Parkinson disease: the TEMPO study. *Arch Neurol* 2002;59:1937–43.

Parkinson Study Group. Dopamine transporter brain imaging to assess the effects of pramipexole vs levodopa on Parkinson disease progression. *JAMA* 2002;287: 1653–61.

Rascol O, Brooks DJ, Korczyn AD et al. A five-year study of the incidence of dyskinesia in patients with early Parkinson's disease who were treated with ropinirole or levodopa. 056 Study Group. *N Engl J Med* 2000;342:1484–91.

Rascol O, Goetz C, Koller W et al. Treatment interventions for Parkinson's disease: an evidence based assessment. *Lancet* 2002;359:1589–98.

Stacy M, Bowron A, Guttman M et al. Identification of motor and nonmotor wearing off in Parkinson's disease: comparison of a patient questionnaire versus a clinician assessment. *Mov Disord* 2005;20:726–33.

Stocchi F ,Vacca L, Ruggieri S, Olanow CW. Intermittent vs continuous levodopa administration in patients with advanced Parkinson's disease: a clinical and pharmacokinetic study. *Arch Neurol* 2005;62:905–10.

Swinn LA, James CR, Quinn NP, Lees AJ. *Treatment of Parkinson's Disease with Apomorphine. Shared Care Guidelines*, 5th edn. London: University College London Hospitals NHS Foundation Trust, 2005.

History

During the 1930s, neurosurgeons attempted to relieve Parkinson's disease symptoms by open brain surgery. The observation that hemiplegic stroke relieved Parkinson's disease tremor on the hemiplegic side led to surgery on the motor tract (Table 4.1). Although these operations were successful at controlling tremor, inevitably they led to paralysis of the affected side and were therefore abandoned.

Irving Cooper's remarkable serendipity is worth recounting: he was attempting pedunculotomy for parkinsonism, when bleeding occurred. The operation was abandoned but the patient improved substantially. Cooper had clipped the anterior choroidal artery, the main blood supply to the globus pallidus. Following this, he embarked on a

TABLE 4.1

History of surgery for Parkinson's disease

Operation	Reference
Pyramidal tract	
Pyramidal tractotomy of cervical cord	Putnam 1940
Cerebral cortex excision	Bucy and Buchanan 1932; Klemme 1940
Cerebral peduncle incision	Walker 1952
Basal ganglia	
Caudate nucleus, globus pallidus lesions	Meyers 1942
Anterior choroidal artery ligation, chemopallidectomy, chemothalamotomy	Cooper 1954
Thalamotomy (ventral-intermediate nucleus)	Narabayashi and Ohye 1978
Pallidotomy	Laitinen et al. 1992

series of operations creating lesions within the globus pallidus and thalamus.

Physiological recording in the thalamus established the ventral-intermediate (VIM) nucleus as the source of tremor. Stereotactic thalamotomy became the most frequently performed operation for Parkinson's disease during the early 1960s because of its profound effect on tremor. However, by the mid-1960s, neurosurgery for Parkinson's disease had almost disappeared because of the introduction of levodopa. When the long-term problems with drug therapy, such as dyskinesias and drug-induced 'on/off' fluctuations, became apparent, the merits of neurosurgery were re-evaluated. This was influenced in particular by Laitinen in 1992, when he reported that his results using pallidotomy (surgery on the globus pallidus) over 20 years indicated sustained benefit.

In addition to lesional 'destruction' surgery, neuronal transplantation was attempted during the 1980s and experimental programs continue. More recently, deep brain stimulation using depth electrodes has been introduced.

Which patients require surgery?

Surgery remains a last resort in a small number of patients when all available pharmacological therapy has failed to control symptoms. It has a morbidity of approximately 2% due to strokes and infection and a mortality of about 0.5%, and is an unpleasant experience.

Patients, their relatives and carers need to understand the limit of any benefits from an operation, and that surgery is not a cure. Sometimes patients are inclined to concentrate on an 'apparent' cure, such as surgery, when actually psychosocial concerns and dysfunctional family relationships are the main issues affecting their quality of life.

Surgery will benefit a small number of patients, mostly those with young-onset Parkinson's disease who have had the disease for many years and who have 'on/off' syndromes. For these patients, the operation of choice is deep brain stimulation of the subthalamus to enable a reduction in dopaminergic therapy and control of dyskinesias. Patients with severe resistant unilateral tremor should undergo single-side thalamic stimulation. Unilateral pallidotomy may be a treatment option for those with severe resistant dyskinesias, but the dilemma of what to do about the other side will remain; concomitant surgery with contralateral deep brain stimulation may be possible. Subthalamic lesional surgery requires long-term evaluation before it can be recommended.

Today, most movement-disorder centers have an allied surgical program. It is not yet possible to say with certainty which patients benefit most from surgery and which operations should be performed. Ideally, surgical centers should take part in collaborative trials to evaluate the potential of lesional surgery and compare this older technique with deep brain stimulation.

Lesional surgery

Lesional surgery may be preferred to deep brain stimulation when a simpler procedure without complex follow-up is required, especially when it is suspected that a patient will not attend the necessary follow-up after insertion of a stimulator, or if patients have to travel long distances. In some parts of the world, the prohibitive cost of the stimulator (about US$32 000/£20 000 for hardware and follow-up) may lead to a preference for lesional surgery.

Lesional surgery is performed by stereotaxy (Figure 4.1). Magnetic resonance imaging (MRI) and other neuroimaging methods are

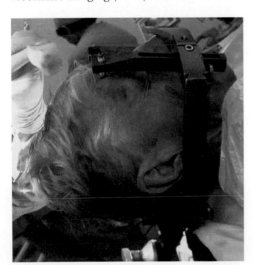

Figure 4.1 Stereotactic frame in place. The frame acts as an external three-dimensional reference for localization of structures within the brain.

insufficient to place a lesion accurately and should be combined with physiological assessment. The patient is therefore woken at the time of lesional placement for physiological stimulation and microelectrode recording. Usually the lesion is created by thermocoagulation; however, cryosurgery is an alternative.

Pallidotomy, a procedure that involves destruction of part of the globus pallidus, is appropriate when there is severe dyskinesia (Table 4.2). Dyskinesias contralateral to the lesion may be greatly alleviated. Pharmacological adjustments are made postoperatively so that 'on' time can be increased. There is a 70% reduction in contralateral tremor and a 30% reduction in activities of daily living score, which allows some patients to return to functional independence.

Bilateral pallidotomy should be avoided because there is a high risk ($\leq 10\%$) of speech and memory disorders. If a second operation is needed on the other side, it should be performed at a later time, and deep brain stimulation should be used in order to avoid permanent side effects.

TABLE 4.2

Pallidotomy

Indications

- Unilateral dyskinesia
- Severe 'on/off' fluctuations (definite levodopa response)
- Age ≤ 75 years
- Drug failure

Contraindications

- Cognitive decline
- Neuropsychiatric problems, e.g. persistent hallucinations, depression
- Previous brain surgery
- Medical problems, e.g. cerebrovascular disease

Thalamotomy, surgery on the VIM nucleus of the thalamus, is the most effective way of controlling tremor. It can be used when tremor is the major disabling feature of Parkinson's disease, and also for essential or ataxic (Holmes') tremor. Deep brain stimulation is the best method of delivery, particularly if a bilateral operation is required. The complication rate is the same as for pallidotomy. Thalamotomy can effectively relieve tremor in 90% of cases, but it should be remembered that tremor is not usually a disabling feature of Parkinson's disease, and thalamotomy has no effect on bradykinesia.

Subthalamotomy is surgery on the subthalamic nucleus, the main outflow tract of the basal ganglia, which is abnormally active in Parkinson's disease. Lesional surgery of the subthalamic nucleus can improve tremor, bradykinesia and rigidity. Its effect can be compared with continuous apomorphine infusion, but it causes less dyskinesia. Care needs to be taken not to provoke dyskinesias or hemiballism. There is ongoing debate as to whether lesional surgery or deep brain stimulation is more effective in inhibiting subthalamic nucleus activity. At present, there is little evidence of long-term efficacy, but rather a suspicion that subthalamotomy may carry a greater complication rate than other lesional surgery performed at the basal ganglia.

Deep brain stimulation

The hypothesis that deep brain stimulation (DBS) (Table 4.3) could inhibit tremor and dyskinesias was proposed when it was found that electrical impulses applied during preoperative testing had this effect. The technology was already available from pain pathway stimulation. Alim Benabid's group in France has pioneered this approach in different movement disorders since 1987. DBS can be used to create electrical depolarization of neurons in any basal ganglia site.

Electrodes are placed in basal ganglia targets using stereotaxy. Initially, wires emerging from the skull are attached to an external stimulator (Figure 4.2). The optimal level of stimulation is achieved when symptoms contralateral to placement are controlled with minimal side effects (such as visual field fluctuation or paresthesias). Several days after the operation an internal stimulator is inserted subcutaneously

TABLE 4.3

Deep brain stimulation

Indications

- Subthalamic stimulation
  - resistant 'on/off' syndrome
  - need for second operation
  - resistant dyskinesias
- Thalamic stimulation
  - tremor: parkinsonian, essential/familial, ataxic (Holmes')
- Pallidal stimulation
  - ? for severe dyskinesia

Contraindications

- Cognitive decline/neuropsychiatric problems
- Severe medical problems
- Patient/carer non-compliance
- Dopa-resistant parkinsonism

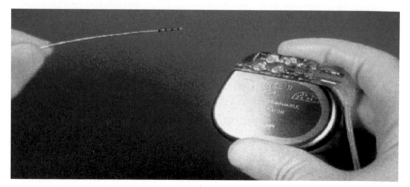

Figure 4.2 Stimulator box and wire.

below the clavicle and connected to a wire tunnelled subcutaneously from the scalp (Figure 4.3). Batteries can last up to 5 years and may be conserved by turning stimulation off at night; the patient can do this using a magnet. Patients undergoing DBS need to be followed up by a team able to monitor and adjust its effects.

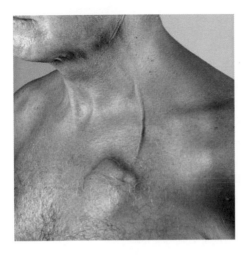

Figure 4.3 Stimulator in place with visible subcutaneous wire.

If bilateral stimulation is required, a second operation can be performed later, although increasingly both operations are performed at the same time. Single stimulator boxes for both hemispheres are now available. Thalamic targets (VIM nucleus) are used for tremor, whether parkinsonian, essential or ataxic (Holmes'), and can provide spectacular results. Tremor will cease within seconds of starting stimulation and reappears quickly on stopping. VIM DBS appears not to be affected by age. The frequency of distal appendicular tremor and greater tremor indicates good control of tremor by VIM DBS. Nevertheless, the subthalamic nucleus is now the preferred target for control of parkinsonian signs. DBS can reverse akinesia, rigidity and tremor but not many axial symptoms. Stimulation of the globus pallidus is more difficult because the target is larger.

A meta-analysis of outcomes from cohorts of patients undergoing DBS of the subthalamic nucleus suggests that dyskinesia is reduced by 69.1% (95% CI: 62–76.2%), the daily 'off' period is reduced by 68.2% (95% CI: 58–79%) and health-related quality of life is improved by 34.5±15.3%. Most studies have excluded patients over the age of 75 years. The most common serious adverse event is intracranial hemorrhage (in 3.9% of patients), and psychiatric sequelae are common. Infection rates have an incidence of 1.6%, and replacement of portions of the device is needed in 4.4% of patients. Clearly, controlled and randomized studies are needed and are currently under way.

Quality of life and mortality. A large randomized study by Deuschl et al. demonstrated that subthalamic neurostimulation resulted in a significant and clinically meaningful improvement in the quality of life of patients under 75 years of age with advanced Parkinson's disease who had severe fluctuations in mobility and dyskinesia. The patients who received neurostimulation had longer periods with less dyskinesia and better-quality mobility.

These changes in motor function also led to improvement in activities of daily living and quality of life (emotional wellbeing, stigma and bodily discomfort). Cognition, mood and overall psychiatric functioning were unchanged. The authors concluded that, in carefully selected patients, neurostimulation of the subthalamic nucleus is a powerful treatment that alleviates the burden of advanced Parkinson's disease. The prospect of an improved quality of life in patients treated with neurostimulation has to be weighed against the risk of complications related to surgery.

A further study by Schupbach and colleagues examined the effect of DBS on mortality in Parkinson's disease, by examining the records of 171 consecutive cases treated by DBS of the subthalamic nucleus. Poor preoperative cognitive function appeared to be a predictive factor for mortality, while survival among patients who underwent surgery was no better than those who did not have the operation.

Nerve-cell transplantation

Attempts to transplant nervous tissue in animals have been made since the 1890s (Table 4.4). Successful transplantation of fetal mesencephalic dopamine neurons was achieved in 1987 (Figure 4.4). Over 500 patients worldwide have now received nerve-cell transplants into the brain.

Aborted 6–10-week-old fetuses are harvested and dissected for midbrain dopamine cells. These are either dispersed in enzymatic solution or injected as clumps of cells. Cells from up to four fetuses are needed for stereotactic injection into eight sites in both hemispheres (caudate and putaminal nuclei).

Patients are given immunosuppressive therapy with ciclosporin and prednisolone (prednisone in the USA) for up to 6 months, although whether this is necessary has not been established. The aim is to

TABLE 4.4

History of nerve-cell transplantation

Operation	Reference
• Unsuccessful transplantation of cortex between cats and dogs	Thompson 1890
• Successful transplantation of fetal rat tissue	Dunn 1917
• Graft survival of rat nervous tissue	May 1955
• Reversal of behavioral changes in rat parkinsonian model	Bjorklund and Stenevi 1979
• Unsuccessful transplantation of adrenal medulla in a human patient with Parkinson's disease	Backlund et al. 1985
• Reversal of monkey parkinsonism	Redmond et al. 1986
• Implantation of fetal mesencephalon in a human patient with Parkinson's disease	Henderson et al. 1991
• Negative results for sham-controlled studies of human fetal transplantation	Freed et al. 2001, Olanow et al. 2003

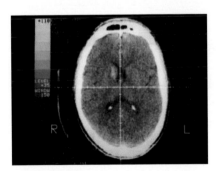

Figure 4.4 Computed tomography scan following transplantation of fetal mesencephalic tissue into the right caudate head of a patient with Parkinson's disease.

restore lost dopamine cells. So far, results indicate that implanted cells can survive, grow and form dendritic connections with host neurons.

There is autopsy evidence of dopaminergic differentiation of these cells, and clinically there have been individual successes, with reversal of motor signs and cessation of dopa drugs. However, in the first controlled trial by Freed et al. in 2001, involving 40 patients

75

randomized to fetal neural transplant or sham surgery, primary outcome measures failed to show any significant differences between the two groups. Furthermore, about 15% of the transplant patients developed severe facial dystonia and disabling 'runaway dyskinesias'.

In a second controlled, double-blind study reported by Olanow et al. in 2003, 34 patients were randomized to either fetal neural transplant with two volumes of donor tissue or sham surgery. Once again primary outcome measures failed to show any significant differences between the two groups, and 56% of transplant patients developed dyskinesias. The authors commented that fetal nigral transplantation cannot be recommended as treatment for Parkinson's disease.

There is hope that cell implantation will replace dopa therapy, but other sources of cells will need to be found if the technique is to become generalized. Immortalized neural stem-cell lines are in development, and porcine fetal cells are undergoing trials but may carry the additional risk of introducing porcine viruses into humans.

The problem remains that even successfully implanted cells may die in the same way as the replaced cells. Research into the rewiring of the human nervous system is ongoing, but it will be decades before a recognized treatment is available.

Glial-cell-line-derived neurotrophic factor

Glial-cell-line-derived neurotrophic factor (GDNF) promotes and supports dopaminergic neuronal cell growth in vitro, and has been shown to have protective effects on dopaminergic neurons in animal models. Several studies in animals have shown that infusion of GDNF into the brain of parkinsonian mice treated with 1-methyl-4-phenyl-1,2,3,6-tetrahydropyridine improved motor function. Postmortem examination of the mice brains showed partial restoration of dopamine in the corpus striatum and dopaminergic fibers in the substantia nigra. However, evidence for the safety and effectiveness of GDNF in humans is lacking.

In 1999, Kordower et al. reported one patient with a 23-year history of Parkinson's disease who developed side effects after intraventricular infusion of GDNF, with no improvement in parkinsonian symptoms and no evidence at postmortem examination of regeneration. However, an open-label phase 1 safety trial in five patients with Parkinson's disease showed improvement in 'off' state and dyskinesias after 1 year, with a 28% increase in putaminal 18-fluorodopa uptake on positron emission tomography scans. However, a subsequent phase 2, double-blind placebo-controlled study in 34 patients with advanced Parkinson's disease failed to show any clinical benefit.

There is also concern that GDNF infusion may cause cerebellar lesions in animal models. Extensive research and clinical trials regarding the mode of delivery, effectiveness and safety of GDNF is required before its use in humans can be recommended.

Retinal-cell transplantation

Retinal pigment epithelium (RPE) is a source of dopamine, and transplantation into the basal ganglia could potentially form a new therapy for Parkinson's disease. In-vitro rat models using a conditioned medium derived from RPE resulted in increased neuritic growth of 78% in striatal neurons, suggesting a potential benefit of RPE transplantation in Parkinson's disease.

One small open-label study in six patients, involving unilateral stereotactic putaminal transplantation of RPE cells attached to biocompatible microcarriers, showed a 34% improvement in the primary outcome measure.

A randomized controlled trial of sham surgery involving RPE is under way.

Spheramine

Spheramine is a cell-based therapy in which normal dopamine-producing cells, such as retinal epithelium, are attached to microcarriers and injected into the basal ganglia. A pilot study involving only six patients with advanced Parkinson's disease, showed a 48% improvement in motor function (on the Unified Parkinson's Disease Rating Scale) and improvements in activities of daily living after 1 year of spheramine therapy; the treatment was well tolerated. Although the results are promising, clinical trials involving larger groups of patients are required.

Key points – neurosurgery

- Surgery is recommended when optimal drug treatment options (including apomorphine therapy) have failed to control symptoms.
- Neurosurgery is an unpleasant experience for the patient; the main complications are strokes and infection.
- For patients with young-onset Parkinson's disease who have had 'on/off' symptoms for many years, the procedure of choice is deep brain stimulation (DBS) of the subthalamic nucleus to reduce dopaminergic therapy and control dyskinesias.
- Lesional surgery is an alternative to DBS for patients unlikely to attend regular follow-up or who have to travel long distances, or in instances where the cost of a stimulator is prohibitive.
- Pallidotomy is appropriate for severe dyskinesia.
- Thalamotomy is the most effective procedure for controlling parkinsonian tremor.
- In the future, nerve-cell transplantation could replace dopaminergic treatment if sources for dopamine cells other than 6–10-week-old fetuses can be found; trials using porcine fetal cells, stem cells that generate dopamine and other such cells (e.g. retinal cells) are under way.

Key references

Backlund EO, Granberg PO, Hamberger B et al. Transplantation of adrenal medullary tissue to striatum in parkinsonism. First clinical trials. *J Neurosurg* 1985;62:169–73.

Benabid AL, Deuschl G, Lang AE et al. Deep brain stimulation for Parkinson's disease. *Mov Disord* 2006;21(suppl14):S168–70.

Benabid AL, Pollak P, Louveau A et al. Combined (thalamotomy and stimulation) stereotactic surgery of the VIM thalamic nucleus for bilateral Parkinson's disease. *Appl Neurophysiol* 1987;50:344–6.

Bjorklund A, Stenevi U. Reconstruction of the nigrostriatal dopamine pathway by intracerebral nigral transplants. *Brain Res* 1979;177:555–60.

Brundin P. GDNF treatment in Parkinson's disease: time for controlled clinical trials? *Brain* 2002;125:2149–51.

Bucy PC, Buchanan DN. Athetosis. *Brain* 1932;55:479–92.

Burton EA, Glorioso JC, Fink DJ. Gene therapy progress and prospects: Parkinson's disease. *Gene Ther* 2003;10:1721–7.

Cooper IS. Surgical alleviation of Parkinsonism: effects of occlusion of the anterior choroidal artery. *J Am Geriatr Soc* 1954;2:691–718.

Cooper IS. 20-year followup study of the neurosurgical treatment of dystonia musculorum deformans. *Adv Neurol* 1976;14:423–52.

Cooper IS, Riklan M. Cryothalamectomy for abnormal movement disorders. *St Barnabas Hosp Med Bull* 1962;1:17–23.

Deuschl G, Schade-Brittinger C, Krack P et al. A randomized trial of deep-brain stimulation for Parkinson's disease. *N Engl J Med* 2006;355:896–908.

Dunn EH. Primary and secondary findings in a series of attempts to transplant cerebral cortex in the albino rat. *J Comp Neurol* 1917; 27:565–82.

Freed CR, Greene PE, Breeze RE et al. Transplantation of embryonic dopamine neurons for severe Parkinson's disease. *N Engl J Med* 2001;344:710–19.

Grondin R, Zhang Z, Yi A et al. Chronic, controlled GDNF infusion promotes structural and functional recovery in advanced parkinsonian monkeys. *Brain* 2002;125:2191–201.

Henderson BT, Clough CG, Hughes RC et al. Implantation of human fetal ventral mesencephalon to the right caudate nucleus in advanced Parkinson's disease. *Arch Neurol* 1991;48:822–7.

Klemme RM. Surgical treatment of dystonia, paralysis agitans and athetosis. *Arch Neurol Psychiatry* 1940;44:926.

Kordower JH, Emborg ME, Bloch J et al. Neurodegeneration prevented by lentiviral vector delivery of GDNF in primate models of Parkinson's disease. *Science* 2000;290:767–73.

Kordower JH, Palfi S, Chen EY et al. Clinicopathological findings following intraventricular glial-derived neurotrophic factor treatment in a patient with Parkinson's disease. *Ann Neurol* 1999;46:419–24.

Laitinen LV, Bergenheim AT, Hariz MI. Leksell's posteroventral pallidotomy in the treatment of Parkinson's disease. *J Neurosurg* 1992;76:53–61.

Madrazo I, Leon V, Torres C et al. Transplantation of fetal substantia nigra and adrenal medulla to the caudate nucleus in two patients with Parkinson's disease. *N Engl J Med* 1988;318:51.

May RM. Cerebral transplantation in mammals. *Transplantation Bull* 1955;2:62.

Meyers R. The modification of alternating tremors, rigidity and festination by surgery of the basal ganglia. *Res Publ Ass Res Nerv Ment Dis* 1942;21:602–65.

Narabayashi H. Surgical approach to tremor. In: Marsden CD, Fahn S, eds. *Movement Disorders*. London: Butterworth Scientific, 1982:292–9.

Narabayashi H, Ohye C. Parkinsonian tremor and nucleus ventralis intermedius of the human thalamus. *Prog Clin Neurophysiol* 1978;5:165–72.

Olanow CW, Goetz CG, Kordower JH et al. A double-blind controlled trial of bilateral fetal nigral transplantation in Parkinson's disease. *Ann Neurol* 2003;54: 403–14.

Putnam TJ. Treatment of unilateral paralysis agitans by section of the lateral pyramidal tract. *Arch Neurol Psychiatry* 1940;44:950–76.

Redmond DE, Sladek JR Jr, Roth RH et al. Fetal neuronal grafts in monkeys given methylphenyltetra-hydropyridine. *Lancet* 1986;1: 1125–7.

Schupbach MW, Welter ML, Bonnet AM et al. Mortality in patients with Parkinson's disease treated by stimulation of the subthalamic nucleus. *Mov Disord* 2007;22:257–61.

Stover NP, Bakay RA, Subramanian T et al. Intrastriatal implantation of human retinal pigment epithelial cells attached to microcarriers in advanced Parkinson's disease. *Arch Neurol* 2005;62:1833–7.

Thompson WG. Successful brain grafting. *N Y Med J* 1890;51:701–2.

Walker AE. Cerebral pedunculotomy for the relief of involuntary movements. II. Parkinsonian tremor. *J Nerv Ment Dis* 1952;116:766–75.

Other therapies and support

A multidisciplinary approach is an absolute requirement for optimal care of the parkinsonian patient. Early on, the main requirement is for information and counseling. In the later stages of the disease, coordination of the various agencies involved in care is often difficult and, as time passes, additional agencies will have to be accessed by the treating physician (Table 5.1).

At diagnosis

Many patients will not be disabled at the time of diagnosis. It is best to break the bad news of a patient's diagnosis in the presence of their spouse, partner or other family members. Often, little information is retained and it is necessary to meet again within 2–3 weeks, when the patient's initial shock has subsided. Reinforcing the diagnosis and the steps made to confirm it should be followed by provision of information

---

TABLE 5.1

Agencies and professionals involved in the care of the parkinsonian patient

- Carer support network
- Family practitioner, geriatrician or neurologist
- Community- or hospital-based therapist, e.g. physiotherapist, speech therapist, occupational therapist, dietitian
- Specialist nurse, e.g. continence nurse, specialist nurse in Parkinson's disease
- Community (district) nurse
- Psychiatrist, psychologist, specialist counselor (e.g. sex therapist)
- Pharmacist
- Local hospital (acute admission)
- Nursing home, if home care is impossible

and advice. Many patients find the support offered by organizations such as the Parkinson's Disease Society helpful (see Useful addresses, page 120). A Parkinson's disease nurse specialist (PDNS) can spend more time with the patient and can offer telephone support. Some patients may need specialist counseling to help them to come to terms with the diagnosis.

Parkinson's disease nurse specialist. The PDNS is a key and essential member of any team dealing with the management of this condition. The PDNS is skilled in patient and carer assessment, differential diagnosis of Parkinson's disease and appropriate drug treatment, medicines management and communication. The role of the PDNS in the care of patients with Parkinson's disease has been reported in three randomized controlled trials (RCTs), although the methodology of these studies has varied widely. The studies reported that PDNS care allowed a swift implementation of good clinical practice for Parkinson's disease, including home visits, and a high rate of patient satisfaction.

Ongoing support

In the early stages, the main focus is often on drug therapy. This should be initiated following specialist advice, but the family physician or PDNS may provide continuing supervision provided there is good liaison with the specialist (neurologist or geriatrician). Therapists have a useful role at all stages of the disease and should work as part of the multidisciplinary team.

Physiotherapists can advise on exercise, gait supervision and strategies for dealing with falls. Walking aids are usually unhelpful, but when falls and fear of falling emerge walking sticks are often adopted. Wheeled delta frames with brakes are better than static frames and allow fluent walking movement when falls become a problem. Despite this, some patients will need a wheelchair outside the home. However, early use of a wheelchair may indicate an alternative diagnosis.

The role of physiotherapy in Parkinson's disease has been examined to a reasonable extent in randomized trials, although a robust evidence base is still lacking. In a Cochrane review of data from 11 randomized trials, four reported a significant improvement in a total of 280 patients after physiotherapy that was directed to the limbs and trunk for 8–30 hours over 3–52 weeks.

Other studies have addressed small numbers of patients only; for example, one randomized trial evaluated 8 patients in a 16-week aerobic exercise program. In another, 88 patients were randomized to the Alexander Technique, massage or a control group. Significant improvements were reported in outcome measures in treated patients versus controls at 6 months.

Physiotherapy in Parkinson's disease is currently recommended to educate patients about gait, initiation of movement and balance, as well as providing advice on safety within the home environment. As such, these interventions are very useful as the condition advances and balance problems, along with fear of falling, become apparent.

Speech therapists can advise on speech exercises and can encourage communication if patients are ignored or feel left out of conversations. In the later stages of disease, speech and language therapists may need to advise on swallowing difficulties, as well as food composition and consistency. If choking is a problem, liquids may be thickened and food homogenized.

The evidence base of efficacy for speech and language therapy (SALT) is limited by the small numbers of patients included in trials: three RCTs have evaluated a total sample of 63 patients. One study investigated the use of Lee Silverman Voice Treatment (LSVT), a speech therapy program comprising 16 1-hour sessions, which was developed in North America with the aim of restoring oral communication in patients with Parkinson's disease. The majority of positive outcomes reported after SALT involve the use of LSVT.

Occupational therapists should be involved if there is difficulty with daily living activities. Adaptation of the home is often necessary when the patient becomes more disabled. For example, ramps and widened doorways will allow wheelchair access, and a shower, rather than a bath, will allow the patient to sit on a stool and wash.

Occupational therapists assess the safety of homes, particularly when the patient is prone to falling. Grab-rails can be fitted, sharp corners protected, and patients can wear hip protectors to prevent hip fractures. Social services may need to be involved to make such changes and to assess the need for financial assistance.

There has been one Cochrane review of the efficacy of occupational therapy in a total of 84 people in two randomized parallel-group trials; no RCTs have been reported using occupational therapy. One trial reported continued maintenance of the Barthel index score (a measure of activities of daily living) over a 1-year period in patients who received occupational therapy.

Carers. Often the brunt of care falls on a patient's spouse or partner. Additional help may be needed to assist the patient with dressing, toileting or bathing. Consultations with the patient should include the carer, with attention given to the carer's mental and physical health and to whether additional support is needed.

Patients who hallucinate or have dementia often provoke social crises and cries for help from carers. Hallucinations may be temporary and related to excessive drug treatment, but often presage cognitive decline with memory difficulties and disorientation. These are the most difficult problems for patients with Parkinson's disease and their carers, and occur in at least 30% of cases. Swift action is required, and the availability of a PDNS is often invaluable.

The first step is to rationalize drug treatment, removing those drugs that are least effective or most likely to cause hallucinosis. Therapy with levodopa plus a decarboxylase inhibitor is often the best policy. Neuroleptics that may aggravate parkinsonism should be avoided.

Support from nurses and social services is vital in keeping patients at home as long as possible, because admission to hospital in this situation may further aggravate decline. Despite this, patients with dementia frequently cannot be managed at home and will need to be admitted to a nursing home, either for respite care or on a permanent basis. Demented patients who are prone to wander may need a locked facility.

Palliative care

The palliative phase of Parkinson's disease is now recognized, and indicates a stage of disease when drugs are no longer well tolerated, the patient is an unsuitable candidate for surgery and there is considerable comorbidity. However, the need for palliative care in Parkinson's disease does not mean an imminent end of life. In the UK, an 'End of Life' initiative has been set up by the Department of Health to train healthcare professionals in the palliative needs and care of patients.

Diet

A healthy diet is recommended, with attention to overall nutrition and roughage. In the early stages of the disease, eating plenty of fruit and vegetables should be encouraged to stimulate a sluggish bowel. Advice from a dietitian may be needed if a patient's nutritional intake is thought to be poor. An early warning sign is afforded when the patient takes longer than the carer to complete meals and does not finish meals. It may be necessary to liquidize food and to provide dietary supplements.

Constipation can be distressing and high-residue diets may make matters worse. Lactulose or other osmotic laxatives are first-line treatment. They will make stools softer but may lead to incontinence. Bowel stimulation using senna can be useful, but more powerful drugs, and eventually suppositories and micro-enemas, may be needed. A recent double-blind placebo-controlled trial reported good efficacy for Movicol® in the treatment of constipation in patients with Parkinson's disease.

Patients often ask how food interferes with drug treatment. In theory, a large protein intake competes with levodopa absorption and thereby prevents the drug's action, but significant dietary changes are not usually required. Even without drug treatment patients often feel worse in the afternoon, which may be due, in part, to a fall in blood pressure after a large meal at lunchtime. If there appears to be a clear-cut relationship between eating large meals and patient deterioration, then changes such as eating more frequent, smaller meals may help. Patients should not restrict their total protein intake, and the overall aim should be to achieve a well-balanced diet.

Bladder symptoms

Bladder symptoms are significant in 50% of patients. In men, symptoms mimic prostatism, although without flow disturbance or postmicturition dribble. In elderly men, symptoms are often a result of both Parkinson's disease and prostatic hypertrophy.

Transurethral resection of the prostate may lead to incontinence, so urodynamic studies and a careful assessment by the urologist are required before this operation is considered.

Treatment with anticholinergics, such as oxybutynin, 2.5 mg twice daily, can relieve urgency and frequency. However, the symptoms may be resistant in later disease and these drugs can cause side effects such as confusion, dry mouth and aggravation of prostatic outflow problems.

It is necessary to rule out additional urinary infection before any treatment. Antidiuretic hormone taken before going to bed at night may relieve nocturnal incontinence or frequency.

A continence nurse will be able to give invaluable advice and will provide continence pads and other appropriate items.

Skin care

Although skin problems related to parkinsonism are common, patients rarely complain about them. Seborrheic dermatitis may cause crusting of the scalp and can be treated with antifungal preparations. Skin lesions may be treated with combination creams that contain antifungals and hydrocortisone. Episodic sweating can be troublesome and is not easily treated, though anticholinergics such as benzhexol may be tried. Drug rashes are not uncommon, particularly with the use of dopamine agonists, and may necessitate withdrawal of the offending drug.

Sexual problems

Sexual problems are not uncommon and are usually the concern of male patients. Early-onset erectile dysfunction may indicate an alternative diagnosis, such as multiple-system atrophy, but also occurs in parkinsonism. Sexual problems can also result from relationship dysfunction (e.g. caused by fear of illness), apathy as part of cognitive decline or inappropriate sexual arousal as a result of drug treatment (particularly dopamine agonists and apomorphine). Alternatively, neuropsychiatric problems as a result of cognitive decline and drug treatment can lead to delusional beliefs regarding spousal infidelity, which may not respond to changes in drug treatment, cognitive therapy or atypical neuroleptics.

Erectile dysfunction, if proven to be the cause of sexual difficulties (i.e. if early-morning erections fail), can be treated with sildenafil in the usual way, assuming there is no medical contraindication or significant hypotension, and provided there has been full discussion with the patient's partner.

Key points – other therapies and support

- Early in the course of the disease, patients most need clear information, advice and counseling.
- Multidisciplinary therapy and input from a Parkinson's disease nurse specialist should be available to all patients at all stages of the disease.
- Physiotherapy is particularly useful at a stage when balance problems become obvious.
- In early Parkinson's disease, patients should be encouraged to eat plenty of fruit and vegetables to stimulate a sluggish bowel.
- Although a large protein intake may compete with levodopa absorption, patients should not restrict their total protein intake.
- Hallucinations often presage cognitive decline with memory difficulties and disorientation, the most difficult problems for both patients and carers; drugs that are most likely to cause hallucinosis should be withdrawn immediately.
- Bladder symptoms, sleep problems and sexual problems are common, and need to be addressed.
- Skin problems are common, but patients do not often complain of them; drug rashes may necessitate withdrawal of the offending agent.
- Patients and carers should be given the chance to discuss end-of-life issues at the appropriate time with suitably trained professionals.

Key references

Baja NPS, Clough CG. Non-motor aspects of idiopathic Parkinson's disease. *Curr Med Lit Parkinson's Disease* 2001;3:1–6.

Chaudhuri KR, Healy D, Schapira AH. Non-motor symptoms of Parkinson's disease: diagnosis and management. *Lancet Neurol* 2006;5:235–45.

Deane KHO, Ellis-Hill C, Playford ED et al. Occupational therapy for Parkinson's disease. *Cochrane Database Syst Rev* 2001, issue 2. CD002813. www.thecochranelibrary.com

Deane KHO, Jones D, Ellis-Hill C et al. Physiotherapy for patients with Parkinson's disease: a comparison of techniques. *Cochrane Database Syst Rev* 2001, issue 1. CD002815. www.thecochranelibrary.com

Deane KHO, Whurr R, Playford ED et al. Speech and language therapy versus placebo or no intervention for dysarthria in Parkinson's disease. *Cochrane Database Syst Rev* 2001, issue 2. CD002812. www.thecochranelibrary.com

Deane KHO, Whurr R, Playford ED et al. Speech and language therapy for dysarthria in Parkinson's disease: a comparison of techniques. *Cochrane Database Syst Rev* 2001, issue 2. CD002814. www.thecochranelibrary.com

Eichhorn TE, Oertel WH. Macrogol 3350/electrolyte improves constipation in Parkinson's disease and multiple system atrophy. *Mov Disord* 2001;16:1176–7.

Jarman B, Hurwitz B, Cook A et al. Effects of community based nurses specialising in Parkinson's disease on health outcome and costs: randomised controlled trial. *BMJ* 2002;324:1072–5.

MacMahon DG, Thomas S. Practical approach to quality of life in Parkinson's disease: the nurse's role. *J Neurol* 1998;245(suppl 1):S19–22.

Quinn NP, Koller WC, Lang AE, Marsden CD. Painful Parkinson's disease. *Lancet* 1986;1:1366–9.

Stallibrass C, Sissons P, Chalmers C. Randomized controlled trial of the Alexander technique for idiopathic Parkinson's disease. *Clin Rehabil* 2002;16:695–708.

End of Life Care Programme, UK www.endoflifecare.nhs.uk/eolc

Long-term complications develop in virtually all patients taking continued levodopa therapy. Although levodopa is the most effective drug for the treatment of Parkinson's disease, the initial benefit begins to diminish over time with dyskinesias and fluctuations in motor response. It is likely that two factors determine the development of fluctuations and dyskinesias (Figure 6.1):

- disease severity
- chronic pulsatile stimulation of postsynaptic dopamine receptors by the use of dopaminergic drugs with a short half-life.

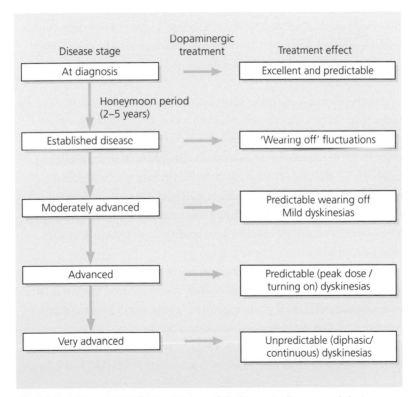

Figure 6.1 The stages of progression of Parkinson's disease and their relationship to motor complications.

Motor fluctuations

Initial treatment with levodopa will reverse parkinsonian symptoms consistently during the day without fluctuations. This occurs despite its short plasma half-life (2–3 hours), and presumably reflects the ability of nigrostriatal dopaminergic neurons to store dopamine before its release into the synapse. Coadministration of a decarboxylase inhibitor, such as carbidopa or benserazide, prevents metabolism of levodopa to dopamine in the bloodstream. These drugs do not cross the blood–brain barrier, and so dopa is decarboxylated to dopamine within the neurons without rate limitation.

Within 2–3 years, most patients begin to experience fluctuations (Table 6.1).

Reversal of parkinsonism correlates with the level of levodopa in the bloodstream. One factor underlying the development of fluctuations is the progressive fallout of dopamine neurons within the striatum, which leads to a reduced capacity for dopamine storage: levodopa arriving in the neuron is metabolized immediately to dopamine and released into the synapse.

Another factor is pharmacokinetic: plasma levels of levodopa become increasingly erratic due to variable absorption from the stomach and duodenum (involving some dietary interaction), together with a greater capacity for levodopa metabolism in the periphery. If low doses of combination therapy are used, decarboxylase may not be blocked effectively: carbidopa, 75 mg daily, is required. Of more importance is the peripheral O-methylation of dopa by catechol-O-methyl transferase to 3-O-methyl-dopa, an inactive metabolite that does not cross the blood–brain barrier (see Figure 3.2).

Fluctuations become increasingly unpredictable over a period of years and are difficult to relate to dopa dosage. 'Dose failures' may be related to the recently described phenomenon of 'internalization' of dopamine receptors, so that drugs become ineffective for a period. Patients are significantly disabled and find it hard to plan their lives, not knowing whether they will be mobile ('on') or frozen ('off'). 'On/off' syndrome becomes the focus of their lives and is a challenging problem for clinicians. Its appearance is related to the severity of disease and the underlying death of dopaminergic neurons.

TABLE 6.1

Types of fluctuation

Long-duration motor fluctuations

- Dose-related early-morning worsening
- End–start dose failure (the drug fails to work sufficiently soon after administration, and/or its effects wear off before the next dose)
- 'On/off' fluctuations
- Circadian or diurnal fluctuations (good response to levodopa in the morning but worsening response in the evening)
- Yo-yo movements (unpredictable)
- Postprandial worsening (following a high carbohydrate/protein meal)

Short-duration fluctuations (occur late in disease)

- Motor blocks, e.g. 'freezing' of gait
  - 'on/off' related
  - unpredictable
- Kinesia paradoxica (sudden relief from parkinsonism in response to stressful stimuli)

Unclassified fluctuations

- Premenstrual worsening (mechanism unclear)
- Late motor deterioration after prolonged levodopa withdrawal (up to 2 weeks later)
- Transient worsening after each dose of levodopa

Dyskinesias

Dyskinesias are hyperkinetic states mostly seen in patients with levodopa-treated Parkinson's disease. In the early stage of the disease, these states are often not noticed by patients and are a good sign of dopa-responsiveness. A large body of research in animal models suggests that dyskinesias arise from alteration of dopaminergic tone in the denervated striatum, together with delivery of treatment by non-physiological pulsatile stimulation of dopamine receptors leading to cellular adaptations such as activation of transcription factors and alteration of downstream gene expression such as the immediate early genes.

Dyskinesias may be related to 'off' or 'on' periods, but as the disease advances they become a continuum and difficult to classify. 'Peak-dose' dyskinesias are the most common. They involve choreic or ballistic movements, and may be associated with a variety of non-motor symptoms such as pain, mood alterations and cognitive changes. Dyskinesias may be socially unacceptable to carers, while patients may prefer to be dyskinetic when 'on'. Most dyskinesias progress and may lead to a reduced quality of life and weight loss. Reducing dopaminergic drugs will diminish dyskinesia, but may lead to a return of Parkinson's disease symptoms. Smaller doses of dopa given more frequently, or a combination of the drug with a dopamine agonist, may help, but problems are likely to reappear (Table 6.2). The findings of a large number of preclinical and clinical studies indicate that continuous dopaminergic stimulation may be the most desirable way to combat dyskinesias.

TABLE 6.2

Management strategies for fluctuations and dyskinesias

Type of fluctuation	Management
Suboptimal peak response / no 'on' period (suboptimal response at peak effect time)	• Increase levodopa dose • Add COMT inhibitor, e.g. entacapone • Add dopamine agonist
Early-morning dystonia	• Late-evening or nighttime dose of controlled-release levodopa or long-acting dopamine agonist
'Wearing off'	• Shorten dosage interval • Pre-meal (up to 60 minutes) levodopa • Dispersible levodopa • COMT inhibitor • Dopamine agonist (short- or long-acting) • Controlled-release levodopa (best used before sleep) • Selegiline

CONTINUED

TABLE 6.2 (CONTINUED)

Management strategies for fluctuations and dyskinesias

Type of fluctuation	Management
Unpredictable 'on/off'	• Combination therapy with levodopa and dopamine agonist • Return to fewer doses of levodopa and combine with intermittent injections or continuous subcutaneous apomorphine • Dietary distribution of protein (small snacks and one large evening meal)
Freezing	
'Off' related	• Increase dopaminergic therapy • Apomorphine (rescue injections)
Random	• Sensory cues • Avoid selegiline
Anxiety related	• Anxiolytics, e.g. amitriptyline

Timing of dyskinesia	Management
Peak dose (usually choreic)	• Reduce individual levodopa dose • Frequent smaller doses, unchanged total • Addition of long-acting dopamine agonist • Consider surgery
'Beginning' or 'end' dose	• Soluble levodopa before meals • COMT inhibitors
Diphasic dyskinesias	• Apomorphine infusion • Add cabergoline • Consider surgery

COMT, catechol-*O*-methyl transferase.

Dementia

Dementia is an important cause of comorbidity in parkinsonism; when cognition declines, mortality increases. Dementia is a bad sign and will often lead to the breakdown of support networks. Patients who are confused and hallucinating become difficult to manage at home and are frequently admitted to nursing homes. At this stage, life expectancy may be only 1–2 years.

Estimation of the incidence of dementia has proved difficult. Most parkinsonian patients have minor cognitive problems that are not apparent to spouses or relatives; 90% have deficits in frontal lobe tests, such as shifting sets (Wisconsin card sorting test). This reflects a rigidity of thought that may be apparent premorbidly for several years.

Characteristically, patients have difficulty 'changing their mind' and slowness of thought, with impairment of central reaction times. This can lead to a false estimation of cognitive function unless time is spent carefully assessing patients.

Global intellectual decline (dementia) is usually a feature of parkinsonism in the elderly, with more than 30% of patients over 70 years affected. Memory disturbance may be a warning sign, although younger patients may complain of short-term memory problems for many years. This may be due in part to drug therapy, particularly with anticholinergics, or to depression.

Hallucinosis is particularly worrying and often presages dementia (Table 6.3).

TABLE 6.3

Stages of hallucination in Parkinson's disease

Stage	Type
1	Vivid dreams (possibly predictive for development of florid hallucinations)
2	Preserved insight (seeing familial figures, deceased pets/relatives)
3	Perceived as real (threatening/frightening visual hallucinations, rarely acoustic)

Excessive dopaminergic therapy or anticholinergic drugs can cause hallucinosis in the early stages of disease, but later hallucinosis may occur without drugs and is difficult to control. Often the next stage involves confusional episodes characterized by disorientation. Dementia associated with Parkinson's disease has been termed subcortical, indicating predominant memory disorders, bradyphrenia and disorientation. This is in contrast to Alzheimer's disease, in which language difficulties and other cortical problems such as dyspraxia are predominant (Table 6.4). The distinction, however, is largely theoretical and is not substantiated by postmortem studies.

TABLE 6.4

Differences between parkinsonian dementia, dementia with Lewy bodies (DLB) and Alzheimer's disease

Feature	Parkinsonian dementia	DLB	Alzheimer's disease
Parkinsonian motor syndrome			
Presentation	Early	Late	Late
Disease course	Progressive	Progressive	Progressive
Response to levodopa	Sensitive	Waning response	No response
Dementia			
Presentation	Late	Early	Presenting feature
Features	Memory loss Disorientation Hallucinations	Hallucinations Disorientation Memory loss	Memory loss Dysphasia Dyspraxia Disorientation
Response to cholinergic therapy			
	Possibly beneficial (under investigation)	Possibly improves behavior	Helps memory for first year

The cause of parkinsonian dementia is unclear. Autopsy studies have indicated a substantial contribution from Alzheimer-type pathology. Lewy bodies in the substantia nigra lead to a parkinsonian motor syndrome in life, and it is thought that they spread into the cortex and cause hallucinosis (occipital and temporal cortex) and other cognitive problems.

Diffuse Lewy-body disease (now termed 'dementia with Lewy bodies', DLB) can present with parkinsonian characteristics, but cognitive decline and hallucinosis will be early features: 60% of Alzheimer's disease patients have extrapyramidal/parkinsonian signs in the later stages.

Management of dementia is difficult and requires the involvement of a multidisciplinary team. The drug regimen used to treat Parkinson's disease should be kept as simple as possible, with the aim of achieving maximum mobility with minimum psychological disturbance (particularly hallucinosis).

Carers often prefer patients who are less mobile and less confused, because they are easier to care for. Wandering can be a problem; if confused, the patient will need constant supervision. Support for the carer is crucial in this situation and, if it cannot be provided, the patient will need residential care.

Depression and anxiety

Depression and anxiety are common accompaniments of Parkinson's disease ($\geq 50\%$, 2.7–70% depression, 50–66% anxiety), which may occur with the shock of the diagnosis or later on due to increasing disability. There is also evidence that depression is endogenous, intrinsic to the condition and part of the neurochemical profile.

Depression/anxiety is a marker for dementia in older patients. However, depression must not be mistaken for dementia. Pseudo-dementia can be mistaken for Parkinson's disease dementia. It is important to seek out depressive features and treat with antidepressants (tricyclic drugs or serotonin-reuptake inhibitors) if there is any suspicion of depression. The debate as to the advantages of the various antidepressants is ongoing.

Apathy

A syndrome of apathy distinct from depression, anxiety and fatigue is increasingly recognized in Parkinson's disease. Separate scales have been devised to assess apathy; it is important to recognize this syndrome, which may masquerade as depression.

Psychosis

Psychosis causes gross impairment in reality testing. Psychotic patients evaluate their perceptions abnormally, leading to incorrect interpretation of external reality. Psychosis consists of delusions (false beliefs about external reality) and hallucinations (sensory perceptions in the absence of external stimuli), and has a variety of causes (Table 6.5).

Drug-induced psychosis appears to result from altered function within dopamine projection neurons originating in the ventral tegmental area. Overstimulation of mesencephalic–limbic dopamine receptors causes limbic system dysfunction, leading to psychosis. The management of drug-induced psychosis is outlined in Figure 6.2.

TABLE 6.5

Causes of psychosis in Parkinson's disease

- Dopaminergic drugs
- Dementia related to Parkinson's disease
- Unmasking of underlying schizophrenia
- Development of dementia with Lewy bodies
- Toxic confusional state in Parkinson's disease induced by
  - infection (particularly urinary or upper respiratory tract infections)
  - metabolic/endocrine upset (e.g. diabetic ketoacidosis)
  - malnutrition
  - dehydration
  - sudden withdrawal of dopaminergic drugs

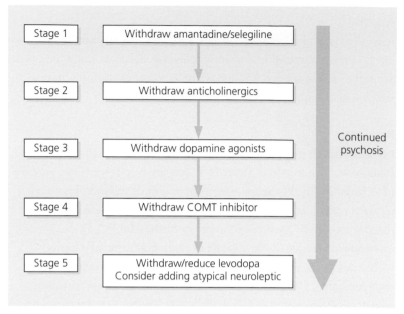

Figure 6.2 Strategy for withdrawing dopaminergic drugs in patients with drug-induced psychosis. COMT, catechol-*O*-methyl transferase.

Typical antipsychotic drugs, such as haloperidol or chlorpromazine, antagonize dopamine D_2 receptors and may cause extrapyramidal side effects such as tardive dyskinesias and parkinsonism. Atypical antipsychotics, such as quetiapine and clozapine, appear to control psychosis without significantly compromising motor function and so are more suitable for treating psychosis in Parkinson's disease (Table 6.6). These agents bind more selectively to serotonin and mesolimbic dopamine receptors than they do to striatal dopamine receptors. However, olanzapine may be hazardous and should be avoided, as it may significantly worsen Parkinson's disease even in small doses. Ondansetron, an antiemetic with action at the serotonin receptors, is also useful in some cases.

Sleep disorders

Sleep problems in Parkinson's disease are common and may affect 60–98% of individuals with the disease, both at early and late stages of the disease. Problems range from disease-related difficulties, such as

TABLE 6.6

Features of atypical antipsychotic (neuroleptic) drug treatment in Parkinson's disease

- All should be started at very low doses
- Drowsiness is common due to antihistamine and antiserotonergic action
- Anticholinergics should be withdrawn before use, otherwise delirium may be precipitated
- White blood cell count is mandatory with clozapine (weekly)
- Ondansetron (a novel 5-HT$_3$ antagonist with a potent antiemetic effect) is expensive and may be occasionally useful
- Postural hypotension is a common side effect
- If an atypical neuroleptic, e.g. sulpiride, is used, a compensatory increase in levodopa dose may be required

rapid eye-movement behavior disorders (RBD), sleep-maintenance insomnia, excessive daytime sleepiness (see pages 54–5) and nocturia, to possibly drug-related problems, such as early-morning dystonia and nighttime akinesia.

The cause of restless legs syndrome in Parkinson's disease remains unclear, although it occurs at approximately twice the rate as that in the general population.

Sleep problems are a key determinant of quality of life in Parkinson's disease, and sleep scales that are specific to the disease such as the Parkinson's Disease Sleep Scale (PDSS) or the SCale for Outcomes in PArkinson's disease (SCOPA) are important for regular clinical assessments.

RBD in particular has emerged as an important symptom that may predict the motor diagnosis of Parkinson's disease by years. The condition may cause self or partner injury, as the patient tends to act out violent dreams in REM sleep. The pathophysiology may involve brainstem nuclei, such as the pedunculopontine nucleus and locus ceruleus, which are involved in stage 2 of the disease (by Braak staging; see pages 12–13), with a motor diagnosis being made in stage 3.

Autonomic problems

Autonomic problems occur with increasing frequency in advanced disease, as has been shown in the recently published NMSQuest study. The problems involve the gastrointestinal systems (constipation, dribbling, dysphagia), orthostatic hypotension, excessive sweating or hyperhidrosis, bladder dysfunction such as detrusor muscle hyperactivity and sexual dysfunction.

Sensory problems

Sensory problems associated with the disease mainly comprise pain syndromes and akathisia, usually in the 'off' state.

Key points – long-term complications

- Virtually all patients taking prolonged levodopa experience long-term complications within 2–3 years of treatment.
- Most dyskinesias progress; smaller, more frequent doses of levodopa, or a combination of the drug with a dopamine agonist, may help but problems are likely to reappear.
- Depression should be treated with antidepressants; depression/anxiety is a marker for dementia in older patients.
- Patients who are confused and hallucinating become difficult to manage at home and life expectancy may diminish to 1–2 years.
- Sleep disorders may affect 60–98% of patients with Parkinson's disease; the presence of rapid eye-movement behavior disorder may predict the motor diagnosis by years.
- The cause of death in Parkinson's disease is most commonly a secondary comorbid disorder.

Key references

Aarsland D, Andersen K, Larsen JP et al. The rate of cognitive decline in Parkinson disease. *Arch Neurol* 2004;61:1906–11.

Chaudhuri KR, Martinez-Martin P, Schapira AH et al. International multicenter pilot study of the first comprehensive self-completed nonmotor symptoms questionnaire for Parkinson's disease: the NMSQuest study. *Mov Disord* 2006;21:916–23.

Emre M. Dementia associated with Parkinson's disease. *Lancet Neurol* 2003;2:229–37.

Marsden CD, Parkes JD. 'On-off' effects in patients with Parkinson's disease on chronic levodopa therapy. *Lancet* 1976;1:292–6.

Playfer JR, Hindle JV, eds. *Parkinson's Disease in the Older Patient*. London: Arnold, 2001:215–38.

Tanner CM, Aston DA. Epidemiology of Parkinson's disease and akinetic syndromes. *Curr Opin Neurol* 2000;13:427–30.

Sato K, Hatano T, Yamashiro K et al. Prognosis of Parkinson's disease: time to stage III, IV, V, and to motor fluctuations. *Mov Disord* 2006;21: 1384–95.

A variety of etiologies that are not secondary to the idiopathic loss of neurons in the substantia nigra may cause parkinsonian syndromes; they include infections, drugs, toxins and structural lesions. In addition, there are a number of degenerative diseases that have a more complex clinical picture than Parkinson's disease and a poorer response to therapy (Table 7.1). It may be impossible to distinguish idiopathic Parkinson's disease from other parkinsonian syndromes by clinical features alone.

An extensive review of the patient's medical history and diagnostic tests, such as neuroimaging, can aid diagnosis (see Chapter 2).

Drug-induced parkinsonism

This is the most common cause of secondary parkinsonism (see pages 110–14), and is often misdiagnosed as Parkinson's disease, because clinical features may be indistinguishable. It causes rigidity, bradykinesia, tremor and gait disturbance, and may be asymmetrical. Although several medications are associated with secondary parkinsonism (Table 7.2), dopamine-blocking agents (neuroleptics) such as prochlorperazine or chlorpromazine are the most common offending agents, and are often prescribed to the elderly for non-specific complaints such as dizziness. The incidence of drug-induced parkinsonism is estimated to be 15–40% in patients receiving neuroleptics, and its prevalence increases with age.

There is some evidence that patients who develop drug-induced parkinsonism may have subclinical Lewy-body Parkinson's disease, which may be unmasked by dopamine-blocking agents.

The effects of dopamine-blocking agents may be prolonged, and drug-induced parkinsonism may take up to 9 months to disappear. Treatment consists of withdrawal of the offending medication. If drug withdrawal is impractical, patients are given the lowest possible dose or are changed to a new atypical agent, such as clozapine or quetiapine. Anticholinergics may be beneficial; levodopa treatment has not been studied systematically.

TABLE 7.1

Degenerative parkinsonian syndromes

- Corticobasal ganglionic degeneration
- Dementia with Lewy bodies
- Multiple-system atrophy
  - MSA-P (predominance of parkinsonian features)
  - MSA-C (predominance of cerebellar features)
- Progressive supranuclear palsy
- Hereditary degenerative diseases
- Autosomal-dominant cerebellar ataxias
  - Machado–Joseph disease, also called spinocerebellar ataxia type 3 (SCA-3)
- Neuronal brain iron accumulation syndromes
  - type 1 and type 2
  - neuroferritinopathy
  - L-ferritin (*FTL*) gene and pantothenate kinase (*PANK)-2* gene mutations
  - aceruloplasminemia
- Prion disorders
- Hereditary frontotemporal dementias
- Huntington's disease
- Neuroacanthocytosis
- Wilson's disease
- Whipple's disease
- X-linked dystonia–parkinsonism (Lubag)
- Parkinsonism–dementia–amyotrophic lateral sclerosis complex of Guam (an atypical unclassifiable parkinsonism found in people on Guadeloupe)

TABLE 7.2

Drugs that can induce parkinsonism

Inhibitors of dopamine synthesis or precursors of a false neurotransmitter

- α-methyl-paratyrosine
- α-methyldopa

Inhibitors of presynaptic dopamine storage

- Reserpine
- Tetrabenazine

Blockers of postsynaptic D_2 receptors

Neuroleptics

- Phenothiazines
  - prochlorperazine
  - amitriptyline
  - thioridazine
  - promethazine
  - fluphenazine
  - mesoridazine
  - trifluoperazine
  - chlorpromazine
  - thiethylperazine
  - perphenazine
- Butyrophenones
  - haloperidol

- Thioxanthenes
  - thiothixene
- Benzamides
  - metoclopramide
- Dihydroindolone
  - molindone
- Dibenzoxazepine
  - loxapine

Miscellaneous D_2-blocking agents

- Tetrabenazine
- Flunarizine
- Amoxapine

γ-aminobutyric acid agonists

- Sodium valproate

Calcium-channel blocker

- Cinnarizine

Progressive supranuclear palsy

Progressive supranuclear palsy (PSP; Steele–Richardson–Olszewski syndrome) presents with gait disturbance and falls (predominantly backwards) in over 50% of cases, and is a disease of later life. The pathological hallmark is tau protein-positive filamentous inclusions, known as neurofibrillary tangles, in the glia and neurons.

The clinical picture consists of supranuclear gaze palsy, particularly down-gaze with nuchal extension, and predominant truncal extensor rigidity. Varying degrees of bradykinesia, dysphagia, personality changes and other behavioral disturbances, such as a subcortical frontal dementia, coexist.

Eye-movement abnormalities (external ocular movements) are very characteristic but may not be present at disease onset. However, patients rarely die without developing these abnormalities. The external ocular movements consist of square-wave jerks, instability of fixation, slow or hypometric saccades and predominantly down-gaze supranuclear palsy. Most simply, patients are unable to look up or down to command, but vertical eye movements following a target are preserved early on, and doll's eye movement is retained until very late.

Limb rest-tremor is rare but has been reported. The presence of asymmetric signs, in particular rest-tremor, would favor a diagnosis of Parkinson's disease over PSP.

Variants of PSP include progressive dementia resembling Alzheimer's disease, pure akinesia and a parkinsonian phenotype. PSP can be confused with frontotemporal dementia, corticobasal degeneration or Pick's disease. Sophisticated magnetic resonance imaging (MRI) of the brain can distinguish PSP from Parkinson's disease, in that the midbrain tectum and tegmentum atrophy in advanced PSP; in addition, the course of PSP is progressive without significant response to levodopa.

Usually, patients die within 5–10 years because of increasing bulbar problems and immobility.

Multiple-system atrophy

Multiple-system atrophy (MSA) consists of a variable combination of parkinsonism with autonomic, pyramidal or cerebellar symptoms and signs. In the past, patients were categorized as having striatonigral type

(SND) if parkinsonian signs were dominant, olivopontocerebellar type (OPCA) if cerebellar signs predominated and Shy-Drager syndrome if autonomic signs were dominant.

Criteria for diagnosis of MSA were formulated by Quinn in 1989 and 1994 and subsequently by Gilman et al. in 1998. The SND and OPCA variants are now called MSA-P and MSA-C, respectively (Table 7.1), and the use of the term Shy-Drager syndrome is discouraged. The pathological feature of MSA is the glial cytoplasmic inclusions.

The main problem is in differentiating Parkinson's disease from the striatonigral type in which the parkinsonian features of MSA include progressive bradykinesia, rigidity and postural instability, and signs that are usually bilateral. Useful clinical clues include disproportionate anterocollis, truncal dystonia (Pisa syndrome), characteristic sighing and the presence of cold, blue hands. Autonomic failure occurs early in MSA and is more severe than in idiopathic Parkinson's disease.

The response to levodopa is commonly incomplete and benefit usually declines within 1–2 years of treatment.

Urinary symptoms are very common. Urodynamic testing reveals a combination of detrusor hyperreflexia and urethral sphincter weakness, which occur in other conditions such as PSP. Neuroimaging may reveal hypointensity of the putamen or an abnormal cross sign, known as the 'hot cross bun' sign, in the pons.

Dementia with Lewy bodies

In dementia with Lewy bodies (DLB), widespread areas of neocortex as well as brainstem and diencephalic neurons have Lewy bodies. Some patients may have associated neurofibrillary tangles consistent with coincidental Alzheimer's disease.

Parkinsonian DLB may be indistinguishable from Parkinson's disease, but patients with the former have early-onset dementia (progressive cognitive decline interfering with normal social and occupational function) and may have hallucinations, delusions and even psychosis in the absence of dopaminergic therapy.

Clinical criteria for diagnosis were developed in 1996 and updated in 1999. Core features of DLB include fluctuations in cognition and attention, recurrent and persistent visual hallucinations and parkinsonian motor signs. Repeated and early falls and neuroleptic sensitivity can be seen. Rarely, patients develop supranuclear gaze palsy; this may lead to the condition being mistaken for PSP.

Response to levodopa tends not to be as complete as in Parkinson's disease, although some patients do respond. The electroencephalogram recording in DLB may be abnormal with background posterior slowing and frontally dominant burst activity, which is not a feature of Parkinson's disease.

Corticobasal ganglionic degeneration

Corticobasal ganglionic degeneration (CBGD), also known as corticodentato-nigral degeneration with neuronal achromasia, typically presents in the sixth or seventh decade with slowly progressive, unilateral development of tremor, apraxia and rigidity in an upper limb.

The condition is characterized by progressive gait disturbances, cortical sensory loss and stimulus-sensitive myoclonus that results in a jerky, useless hand. A jerky, useless lower extremity is uncommon, but may occur. The latter is known as the alien limb phenomenon and can occur in about 50% of patients. Gait disturbance consists of a slightly wide-based, apraxic gait rather than the typical festinating gait of Parkinson's disease. Patients with CBGD do not benefit from levodopa, and the disease course is relentlessly progressive.

The clinical spectrum of this disorder has been expanded recently to include early-onset dementia and aphasia. Other clinical signs include frontotemporal dementia, and visuospatial and visuoperceptive deficits. MRI reveals focal atrophy, particularly in the parietal areas, and positron emission tomography (PET) scans show an asymmetrical decrease in regional cerebral glucose metabolic rates.

Parkinsonism in young adults

The onset of parkinsonism before the age of 40 years is usually called young-onset parkinsonism. Onset of Parkinson's disease at this age is not rare. When symptoms begin before the age of 20, the term juvenile parkinsonism may be used. Parkinsonism at this early an age typically occurs as a component of a more widespread degenerative disorder or a genetic disorder.

Disorders such as Wilson's disease, Huntington's disease and dentato-rubral-pallidoluysian atrophy should be ruled out by appropriate copper measurements and genetic testing. Often, young-onset Parkinson's disease can remain exquisitely sensitive to levodopa for many years, with concurrent development of increasing dyskinesia. The earlier the onset of Parkinson's disease, the more likely that genetic factors are important, and the greater the need for enquiry into family history.

Dopa-responsive dystonia. Patients with young-onset parkinsonism manifest dystonia, which may respond to dopaminergic drugs. However, there is another entity called dopa-responsive dystonia (Segawa's disease), which usually starts in childhood or adolescence. Dystonia is the predominant phenotypic expression; autosomal dominance is the usual inheritance. Patients have a guanosine triphosphate (GTP)-cyclohydrolase deficiency, the genetic abnormality for which is found on chromosome 14.

The disorder characteristically shows marked diurnal variation, and may start in childhood with an odd and unusual gait. Patients demonstrate an excellent and sustained response to low-dose levodopa. Childhood dystonia or unexplained spastic gait should therefore be given a trial of low-dose levodopa, 100 mg once daily. Some family members may show later-onset parkinsonism.

PET scans demonstrate markedly reduced 6-fluorodopa uptake in patients with young-onset Parkinson's disease, while fluorodopa uptake is normal in patients with dopa-responsive dystonia.

Wilson's disease should be considered in every case of young-onset parkinsonism, because it is treatable and the consequences of non-recognition can be grievous. The most common neurological manifestations include tremor, dystonia, rigidity, dysarthria, drooling and ataxia. A combination of parkinsonism and ataxia is characteristic of neurological Wilson's disease. Tremor typically involves the upper limbs and the head, and rarely the lower limbs; classically, the tremor is coarse, irregular and present during action. Holding the arms forward and flexed horizontally may demonstrate the activity of the proximal muscles (wing-beating tremor).

Kayser–Fleischer rings – rings of brownish-green pigmentation – due to copper deposition in the cornea may be easy to recognize in patients with light-colored irises, and are best appreciated with a careful slit-lamp examination performed by an ophthalmologist.

Almost all patients with neurological features have MRI abnormalities in the basal ganglia. There is a pattern of symmetrical, bilateral, concentric-laminar T2 hyperintensity in the putamen and involvement of the pars compacta of the substantia nigra, periaqueductal gray matter, the pontine tegmentum and the thalamus.

The most useful diagnostic test results are a low serum ceruloplasmin level and a raised 24-hour urinary copper excretion. Slit-lamp examination should be performed looking for Kayser-Fleischer rings (see above). Not all patients have a low ceruloplasmin level because inflammation, infection or oral contraceptive use may cause false elevations. Liver biopsy to show copper deposition remains the gold standard diagnostic test.

Juvenile Huntington's disease is an autosomal-dominant neurodegenerative disorder that typically presents with chorea, difficulty with gait and cognitive problems. However, the Westphal variant of the disease, which affects the young, may resemble parkinsonism.

Eye-movement abnormalities, including apraxia, distinguish juvenile Huntington's disease from Parkinson's disease.

Gene testing for Huntington's disease (which may show a cytosine, adenine and guanine [CAG] expansion greater than 35 trinucleotides) should be performed in all patients with juvenile-onset Parkinson's disease, and in adults with unusual features and cognitive decline.

Hemiparkinsonism hemiatrophy syndrome

Patients with this syndrome have a long-standing hemiatrophy of the body and develop a progressive bradykinesia with dystonic movements around the age of 40 years. Ipsilateral corticospinal tract signs, which are not a feature of Parkinson's disease, may be found. Neuroimaging reveals atrophy of the contralateral hemisphere with compensatory ventricular dilatation.

Neuroacanthocytosis

Neuroacanthocytosis is a rare cause of parkinsonism and typically presents with a hyperkinetic movement disorder, including chorea, tic-like features and polyneuropathy. MRI shows characteristic atrophy of the caudate nucleus and hyperintensity in the putamen on T2-weighted images. Acanthocytes are revealed on a fresh blood smear.

Secondary parkinsonism

The term 'secondary parkinsonism' refers to parkinsonism induced by known agents or factors. In addition to drugs (see page 102; Table 7.2), these include infections, toxins, structural lesions and vascular disease.

Encephalitis lethargica and postencephalitic parkinsonism. From 1919 to 1926 there were several pandemic outbreaks of encephalitis lethargica (von Economo's encephalitis). Patients had headache, fever, somnolence and ophthalmoplegia. After a variable delay, a number of patients developed parkinsonism associated with psychiatric abnormalities, ophthalmoplegia and oculogyric crises. In this condition tremor tends to be less prominent than in Parkinson's disease, and other movement disorders, including dystonia, may be seen. The oculogyric crises, which do not occur in idiopathic Parkinson's disease, are characterized by forceful deviation of the eyes, usually upwards or upwards and laterally. Sometimes obsessional thoughts or fear and anxiety accompany attacks.

Parkinsonism is rarely associated with other forms of viral encephalitis, such as the arboviruses, measles, polio, coxsackie, echo-viruses, herpes simplex, varicella, Japanese encephalitis or western equine encephalitis.

The response of postencephalitic parkinsonism to levodopa is inconsistent and may wane after an excellent improvement or 'awakening'. In a follow-up study of 50 patients, a third continued to benefit, a third showed no response and the remaining patients could not tolerate the drug.

Other infectious etiologies. Neurological complications, including parkinsonism, may occur in patients with acquired immune deficiency syndrome (AIDS). Parkinsonian features may be secondary to AIDS-associated cerebral infections or cerebral infection with human immunodeficiency virus (HIV) alone. Other rare infections have been reported to cause parkinsonism, including fungal infections, *Mycoplasma pneumoniae*, syphilis, Creutzfeldt–Jakob disease, and cryptococcal and cysticercus infections. In this situation it is usually obvious that parkinsonism is part of a more widespread brain disorder and/or there is evidence of central-nervous-system infection (fever, meningism, confusion).

Toxins. Parkinsonism can be caused by a variety of toxins including carbon monoxide, 1-methyl-4-phenyl-1,2,3,6-tetrahydropyridine (MPTP) (Figure 7.1), manganese and cyanide. Manganese toxicity has been linked to welding-related parkinsonism (see page 19). Onset of symptoms may be subacute following toxin exposure, and the course of disease is progressive. MPTP causes a pure motor parkinsonian syndrome that responds well to levodopa. Other toxins produce a more complex parkinsonian syndrome unresponsive to levodopa.

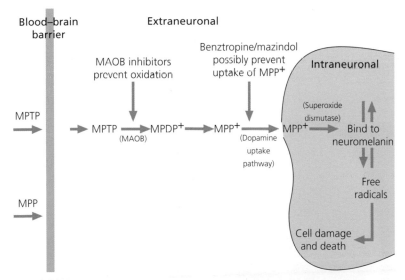

Figure 7.1 The mechanism of action of 1-methyl-4-phenyl-1,2,3,6-tetra-hydropyridine (MPTP) and how it causes parkinsonism. MAOB, monoamine oxidase B; MPDP, 1-methyl-4-phenyl-2,3-dihydropyridine; MPP, 1-methyl-4-phenylpyridine.

Structural lesions that either directly or indirectly affect the basal ganglia may produce parkinsonism. Lesions secondary to hypoxia, hydrocephalus, tumors, vascular disease including strokes and vascular malformations, and demyelinating lesions have been associated with parkinsonism. These are almost always identified on MRI scans.

Hydrocephalus. Patients with hydrocephalus may develop parkinsonian symptoms months or years after initially presenting with hydrocephalus (Figure 7.2), or parkinsonism may develop acutely due to shunt failure, with resolution following shunt revision. Clinically, patients may have tremor, rigidity and bradykinesia.

Normal-pressure hydrocephalus is characterized by the triad of gait difficulty, dementia and urinary incontinence. Poor postural reflexes and flexed posture may also be seen. The hydrocephalus should be treated either by shunting or by shunt revision in the case of malfunction. If parkinsonian symptoms do not respond to shunting, some patients may be sensitive to dopaminergic therapy with a dopamine agonist or levodopa. Normal-pressure hydrocephalus is diagnosed frequently, and many patients undergo shunting without adequate results. This may reflect difficulty in selecting patients who will benefit from treatment: those presenting with gait difficulty alone show the best response, while those with a predominantly cognitive presentation respond poorly and may have a neurodegenerative problem such as Alzheimer's disease.

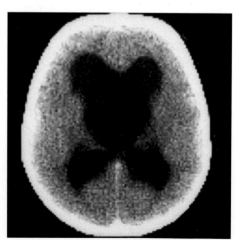

Figure 7.2 Scan of hydrocephalic brain, showing massive dilatation of the cerebral ventricles.

Tumors are a rare cause of parkinsonism. Those associated with parkinsonism occur in several regions of the brain including the striatum, frontal lobe, temporal lobe, parietal lobe, thalamus/hypothalamus, substantia nigra, midbrain and third ventricle. A variety of tumor types have been described, including:

- glioma
- meningioma
- lymphoma
- fibrosarcoma
- metastasis.

Usually patients present with a one-sided, progressive syndrome that does not respond to levodopa. Other signs, such as upper motor neuron signs and a rapidly progressive disease course, will distinguish tumor-related parkinsonism from Parkinson's disease and will determine whether a diagnostic scan is necessary.

Vascular disease is a rare cause of a straightforward parkinsonian syndrome with a variety of clinical presentations. Onset is either acute or subacute, and symptoms (usually bilateral) are those seen in classic Parkinson's disease, including tremor, bradykinesia, rigidity and postural instability. The disease course may be stable from onset or progressive, or may resolve spontaneously. A subgroup of patients may present with predominant lower-extremity symptoms, such as a gait disturbance with minimal upper-extremity symptoms (lower-body parkinsonism), or walking with small steps (marche à petits pas), which is characteristic of vascular disease. Often, additional signs such as spasticity or abnormal plantar reflexes are present.

Post-traumatic parkinsonism. An isolated head injury seldom leads to parkinsonism unless it causes significant brain damage. However, multiple minor head injuries may cause cumulative damage resulting in parkinsonism and dementia, as seen in boxers who have suffered multiple knock-outs (dementia pugilistica). Radiologically, diffuse brain atrophy and a large cavum septum pellucidum, a cavity within the dividing membranes of the lateral ventricles, characterize this condition.

113

Miscellaneous causes. Parkinsonism may occur transiently during alcohol withdrawal. Metabolic causes include hypoparathyroidism with basal ganglia calcifications. There are a few reports of Sjögren's syndrome with associated parkinsonism, but whether parkinsonism is more common in Sjögren's syndrome or the association is coincidental is unclear. Parkinsonian features have been described in central pontine and extrapontine myelinolysis, and in Behçet's disease.

Key points – other parkinsonian syndromes

- It may be impossible to distinguish Parkinson's disease from other parkinsonian syndromes by clinial features alone.
- Progressive supranuclear palsy presents with gait disturbance and falls in later life; asymmetric signs (e.g. rest-tremor) favor a diagnosis of Parkinson's disease.
- Patients with parkinsonian dementia with Lewy bodies have early-onset dementia, and may have hallucinations or psychosis in the absence of dopaminergic therapy.
- Parkinsonism that presents before the age of 20 is more likely to be the result of a widespread degenerative or genetic disorder.
- Drug-induced parkinsonism is the most common cause of secondary parkinsonism.

Key references

Cummings JL. Reconsidering diagnostic criteria for dementia with Lewy bodies. Highlights from the Third International Workshop on Dementia with Lewy Bodies and Parkinson's Disease Dementia, September 17–20, 2003, Newcastle Upon Tyne, United Kingdom. *Rev Neurol Dis* 2004;1:31–4.

Gilman S, Low PA, Quinn N et al. Consensus statement on the diagnosis of multiple system atrophy. American Autonomic Society and American Academy of Neurology. *Clin Auton Res* 1998;8:359–62.

Hughes AJ, Daniel SE, Ben-Shlomo Y, Lees AJ. The accuracy of diagnosis of parkinsonian syndromes in a specialist movement disorder service. *Brain* 2002;125:861–70.

McKeith IG, Galasko D, Kosaka K et al. Consensus guidelines for the clinical and pathologic diagnosis of dementia with Lewy bodies (DLB): report of the consortium on DLB international workshop. *Neurology* 1996;47:1113–24.

McKeith I, Mintzer J, Aarsland D et al.; International Psychogeriatric Association Expert Meeting on DLB. Dementia with Lewy Bodies. *Lancet Neurol* 2004;3:19–28.

Quinn N. Multiple system atrophy – the nature of the beast. *J Neurol Neurosurg Psychiatry* 1989;suppl: 78–89.

Steele JC. Progressive supranuclear palsy. *Brain* 1972;95:693–704.

Wenning GK, Poewe W, eds. Atypical parkinsonian disorders. *Mov Disord* 2005;20 (suppl12):S1–126.

8 Future trends

Although research has helped to develop a range of pharmacological and surgical therapies for Parkinson's disease, we are still unable to cure the disease or slow its progression. In future, the goal of treatment will be prevention and cure, and management strategies will be based on finding a treatable cause (Table 8.1).

Recent evidence suggests that the neurodegenerative process in Parkinson's disease is a final outcome of several interrelated processes:

- oxidative stress from toxic free-radical production
- mitochondrial dysfunction
- accumulation of excitotoxic molecules, such as nitric oxide and oxidative free radicals
- inflammatory changes.

A combination of these processes results in cell death by both necrosis and apoptosis. These depend on external (environmental) and internal (genetic) factors, the balance of which varies from patient to patient.

New medicines in development

Several compounds are being developed that continue to exploit the dopamine pathway but selectively stimulate different dopamine receptors (D_1–D_5). Some compounds, such as ABT-431, are thought to selectively stimulate dopamine D_1 rather than D_2 receptors. Others, such as U-95667E, stimulate D_2 receptors selectively. Preferential stimulation of dopamine receptors may offer control of parkinsonism without dyskinesia.

Neuroprotection remains a key therapeutic target and various strategies are being investigated, including the use of antioxidants, enhancers of mitochondrial function, antiapoptotic agents, glutamate antagonists, anti-inflammatory drugs and anti-protein aggregation drugs. Glutamate, an excitatory amino acid, may lead to overstimulation and cell death in the substantia nigra, so compounds that block glutamate stimulation via N-methyl-D-aspartate receptors are

TABLE 8.1

Future strategies for pharmacological treatment

Restoration of dopamine

- Dopamine creation
- Dopamine conservation
- Selective striatal dopamine-receptor stimulation

Non-dopaminergic modulation

- Newer anticholinergics
- Adenosine A_2 antagonists
- Cannabinoids
- α-adrenoceptor antagonists

Neuroprotective therapy (to slow, halt or reverse progressive neurodegeneration)

- Antiglutamate agents (N-methyl-D-aspartate antagonists), e.g. riluzole, remacemide, amantadine, modafinil, memantine
- Antioxidants, e.g. ascorbic acid, vitamin E, rasagiline
- Anti-apoptosis agents, e.g. selegiline, dopamine agonists, TCH346, CEP-1347
- Mitochondrial enhancers, e.g. coenzyme Q10, creatine
- Anti-inflammatory drugs, e.g. cyclooxygenase (COX-1, COX-2) inhibitors, minocycline
- Trophic factors, e.g. glial-cell-line-derived neurotrophic factor, GPI-1485, GM-1 ganglioside
- Protein aggregate inhibitors, e.g. radicicola, rapamycin, trehalose, small ubiquitin-like modifier (SUMO)-1, valproic acid

under investigation. Riluzole, a glutamate antagonist, was investigated for potential neuroprotective effect in untreated patients, but this trial was stopped because interim analysis showed no effect on disease progression. Remacemide, another proposed neuroprotective agent, has also failed to demonstrate any significant beneficial effect in preliminary clinical trials. Modafinil, used for treating sleepiness, is another drug with antiglutamate action that is under consideration.

A pilot study (referred to as QE2) investigating a possible disease-altering effect of coenzyme Q10 (a fat-soluble vitamin) in a small number of patients with Parkinson's disease suggested a possible beneficial effect at a large dose (1200 mg/day). These results are being studied in a larger trial (QE3). However, the findings of the Neuroprotection Exploratory Trials in Parkinson's Disease (NET-PD), studies run by the US National Institutes of Health to find drugs with the potential to slow the progression of the disease, were discouraging for this compound as it was not considered to be any better than placebo.

Apoptosis causes cell death, and anti-apoptotic agents such as TCH346 and caspase inhibitors have been evaluated and found to be ineffective in slowing down the course of Parkinson's disease. Minocycline, a caspase inhibitor, has been investigated in a NET-PD trial and is not going to be studied any further.

Free-radical production may cause dopamine neuronal degeneration. All of the following may help prevent cell death: 'spin-trap' agents that reduce oxidative stress by scavenging free radicals; agents that chelate iron, such as some forms of apomorphine; or agents that enhance glutathione release. Examples are CU 02-584 and CP1 1189. Alternatively, inhibition of enzymes such as calpain, a calcium-activated proteinase, or caspases (cysteine proteases) may prevent apoptosis.

Protein accumulation appears to be a key feature in the pathogenesis of Parkinson's disease, and agents such as rapamycin, trehalose and small ubiquitin-like modifier (SUMO)-1 appear to prevent protein aggregation. These drugs may be investigated as potential neuroprotective agents.

Gene therapy

The rationale of gene therapy is based on the prospect of producing proteins in situ that will restore dopamine biosynthetic capacity in patients with Parkinson's disease. This involves the delivery of transgenes using various vectors in experimental models of Parkinson's disease. These include genetically modified stem cells differentiated into functioning dopaminergic cells, strategies combining anti-apoptotic action and glial-cell-line-derived neurotrophic factor (GDNF).

Gene therapy can be achieved by:

- genetically modified cell transplantation using immortalized cell lines, e.g. fibroblast or neuroblastoma
- direct in-vivo delivery of viral vectors, e.g. retrovirus ssRNA and adenovirus sDNA
- direct in-vivo delivery of chemically compacted ('naked') DNA.

One trial of human gene therapy has used the expression of glutamic acid decarboxylase to catalyse the production of the inhibitory γ-aminobutyric acid in the subthalamic nucleus. Another trial evaluating neuturin (from the same family of neurotrophins as GDNF) and the aromatic L-amino acid decarboxylase-enhancing gene (with the aim of increasing dopamine production) has also begun.

Key references

Gill SS, Patel NK, Hotton GR et al. Direct brain infusion of glial cell derived neurotrophic factor in Parkinson's disease. *Nat Med* 2003;9:589–95.

Lang AE, Gill S, Patel NK et al. Randomized controlled trial of intraputamenal glial cell line derived neurotrophic factor infusion in Parkinson's disease. *Ann Neurol* 2006;59:459–66.

Tintner R, Jankovic J. Treatment options for Parkinson's disease. *Curr Opin Neurol* 2002;15:467–76.

Update on the management of motor complications in Parkinson's disease. *Mov Disord* 2005;20(suppl 11): S1–56.

Useful addresses

UK

Association of British Neurologists
Ormond House, 27 Boswell Street
London WC1N 3JZ
Tel: +44 (0)20 7405 4060
info@theabn.org
www.theabn.org

**British Association/College of
Occupational Therapists**
106–114 Borough High Street
Southwark, London SE1 1LB
Tel: +44 (0)20 7357 6480
www.cot.org.uk

Carers UK
20–25 Glasshouse Yard
London EC1A 4JT
Advice Line: 0808 808 7777
(Weds/Thurs 10 AM–12 PM; 2–4 PM)
Tel: +44 (0)20 7490 8818
info@carersuk.org
www.carersuk.org

Disabled Living Foundation
380–384 Harrow Road
London W9 2HU
Helpline: 0845 130 9177
(Mon–Fri 10 AM–4 PM)
Tel: +44 (0)20 7289 6111
advice@dlf.org.uk
info@dlf.org.uk
www.dlf.org.uk

**The National Council for
Palliative Care**
The Fitzpatrick Building
188–194 York Way
London N7 9AS
Tel: +44 (0)20 7697 1520
enquiries@ncpc.org.uk
www.ncpc.org.uk

**Parkinson's Disease Non-Motor
Group**
www.pdnmg.com

Parkinson's Disease Society
215 Vauxhall Bridge Road
London SW1V 1EJ
Tel: +44 (0)20 7931 8080
enquiries@parkinsons.org.uk
www.parkinsons.org.uk

**SPRING (Special Parkinson's
Research Interest Group)**
http://spring.parkinsons.org.uk

USA

**American Association of
Neuroscience Nurses**
4700 W Lake Avenue
Glenview, IL 60025
Toll-free: 1 888 557 2266
Tel: +1 847 375 4733
info@aann.org
www.aann.org

American Parkinson Disease Association Inc.
135 Parkinson Avenue
Staten Island, NY 10305
Toll-free: 1 800 223 2732
Tel: +1 718 981 8001
apda@apdaparkinson.org
www.apdaparkinson.org

APDA Young Parkinson's Information and Referral Center
2100 Pfingsten Road
Glenview, IL 60026
Toll-free: 1 800 223 9776
Tel: +1 847 657 5787
info@youngparkinsons.org
www.youngparkinsons.org

LSVT Foundation
(Lee Silverman Voice Treatment)
www.lsvt.org

National Parkinson Foundation
1501 NW 9th Ave, Bob Hope Road
Miami, FL 33136-1494
Toll-free: 1 800 327 4545
Tel: +1 305 243 6666
contact@parkinson.org
www.parkinson.org

The Parkinson Alliance
PO Box 308, Kingston
NJ 08528-0308
Toll-free: 1 800 579 8440
Tel: +1 609 688 0870
www.parkinsonalliance.org

Parkinson's Action Network
1025 Vermont Ave, NW Suite 1120
Washington, DC 20005
Toll-free: 1 800 850 4726
Tel: + 1 202 638 4101
info@parkinsonsaction.org
www.parkinsonsaction.org

Parkinson's Disease Foundation
1359 Broadway, Suite 1509
New York, NY 10018
Toll-free: 1 800 457 6676
Tel: +1 212 923 4700
info@pdf.org
www.pdf.org

Parkinson's Resource Organization
74090 El Paseo, Suite 102
Palm Desert, CA 92260
Toll-free: 1 877 775 4111
Tel: +1 760 773 5628
info@parkinsonsresource.org
www.parkinsonsresource.org

The Parkinson's Web
http://pdweb.mgh.harvard.edu

WEMOVE (Worldwide Education and Awareness for Movement Disorders)
204 West 84th Street
New York, NY 10024
wemove@wemove.org
www.wemove.org

International Association of Physiotherapists in Parkinson Disease Europe
Secretariat, Felicity Handford
Rue W Coppens 6
1170 Watermael Boisfort
Brussels, Belgium
appde@Skynet.be
http://appde.unn.ac.uk
(or contact the European
Parkinson's Disease Association
[below] for more information)

European Parkinson's Disease Association
4 Golding Road
Sevenoaks, Kent TN13 3NJ, UK
Tel/Fax: +44 (0)1732 457 683
lizzie@epda.eu.com
www.epda.eu.com

The Movement Disorder Society
555 East Wells Street, Suite 1100
Milwaukee, WI 53202-3823, USA
Tel: +1 414 276 2145
info@movementdisorders.org
www.movementdisorders.org

Parkinson's Association of Ireland
Carmichael House
North Brunswick Street
Dublin 7
Toll-free: 1 800 359 359
parkinsonsireland@eircom.net
www.parkinsons.ie

Parkinson Association South Africa
Private Bag X36
Bryanston 2021
South Africa
Tel: + 27 (0)11 787 8792
parkins@global.co.za
www.parkinsons.co.za

Parkinson's Australia
Frewin Place
Scullin ACT 2614
Canberra, Australia
Tel: + 61 (0)2 6278 8916
parkinsons.australia@yahoo.com.au
www.parkinsons.org.au

Parkinsons New Zealand
PO Box 10 392, Wellington
New Zealand
Tel: + 64 04 472 2796
Toll-free: 0800 473 4636
info@parkinsons.org.nz
www.parkinsons.org.nz

Parkinson Society Canada
4211 Yonge Street
Suite 316, Toronto
Ontario M2P 2A9, Canada
Toll-free: 1 800 565 3000
Tel: +1 416 227 9700
general.info@parkinson.ca
www.parkinson.ca

Index

What the reviewers say:

concise, well written and illustrated, colourful, informative and factual…
One to dip in and out of, yet small enough to read cover to cover. Buy it
yourself, but be careful your colleagues don't borrow it indefinitely.

On *Fast Facts – Asthma*, 2nd edn, in *Primary Health Care*, 2007

This is a welcome extension to the *Fast Facts* series...
It provides easily accessible information in a user-friendly fashion

On *Fast Facts – Inflammatory Bowel Disease*, 2nd edn, in *Doody's Health Sciences Review*, Aug 2006
(Winner of the BMA Medical Book Award for Gastroenterology, 2006)

perhaps the best source of practical guidance
on infant nutrition for all healthcare staff

On *Fast Facts – Infant Nutrition*, in *Nutrition and Dietetics*, June 2006

This is a book you will want to have

On *Fast Facts – Renal Disorders*,
in *EDTNA/ERCA Journal*, XXXII(1), 2006

the only book available that provides such a concise and
pertinent presentation on bladder cancer and its management

On *Fast Facts – Bladder Cancer*, 2nd edn, in *Doody's Health Sciences Review*, June 2006

I, for one, will make it part of
the mandatory reading for all my
respiratory registrars

On *Fast Facts – Obstructive Sleep Apnea*,
in *Australasian Sleep Association Newsletter*, December 2005

the entire book can be read as a crash course in less than two hours,
yet it does not ignore the complexity of human sexuality

On *Fast Facts – Sexual Dysfunction*, in
Journal of Nervous and Mental Disease, 193(6), 2005

quite simply, a terrific little book...
a fount of evidence-based wisdom

On *Fast Facts – Smoking Cessation*, in *Medical Journal of Australia*, 182(12), 2005

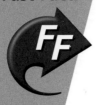
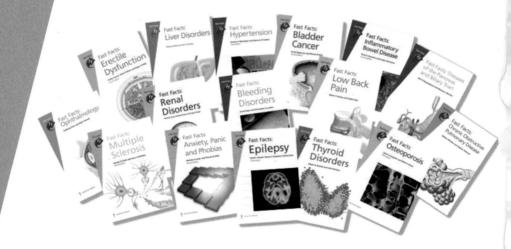